Safe Handling
of Hazardous Drugs
Video Training Program

Luci A. Power, MS, RPh
Senior Pharmacist, Manager
Parenteral Support Services
Department of Pharmaceutical Services
University of California Medical Center
San Francisco, California

James A. Jorgenson, MS, RPh, FASHP
Associate Dean for Clinical Affairs and
Administrative Director for Pharmacy Services
University of Utah
Salt Lake City, Utah

Any correspondence regarding this publication should be sent to the publisher, American Society of Health-System Pharmacists, 7272 Wisconsin Avenue, Bethesda, MD 20814, attention: Special Publishing.

The information presented herein reflects the opinions of the contributors and advisors. It should not be interpreted as an official policy of ASHP or as an endorsement of any product. The information contained in this program, and the companion workbook, are to be used as guidance.

Because of ongoing research and improvements in technology, the information and its applications contained in this text are constantly evolving and are subject to the professional judgment and interpretation of the practitioner due to the uniqueness of each pharmacy's role in compounding sterile preparations and the handling of hazardous drugs. The editors, contributors, and ASHP have made reasonable efforts to ensure the accuracy and appropriateness of the information presented in this document. However, any user of this information is advised that the editors, contributors, advisors, and ASHP are not responsible for the continued currency of the information, for any errors or omissions, and/or for any consequences arising from the use of the information in the document in any and all practice settings. Any reader of this document is cautioned that ASHP makes no representation, guarantee, or warranty, express or implied, as to the accuracy and appropriateness of the information contained in this document and will bear no responsibility or liability for the results or consequences of its use.

Acquisitions Editor & Producer: Hal Pollard
Senior Editorial Project Manager: Dana Battaglia
Project Manager & Producer: Peter Cantor
Instructional Designer: Holly O'Hare, ICS Learning Group
Film Director: Frank Lama, ICS Learning Group
Production: Johnna Hershey, Carol Barrer
Package Design: Armen Kojoyian

ISBN: 1-58528-139-5

Table of Contents

Continuing Education

HOW TO EARN CONTINUING PHARMACY EDUCATION (CE) CREDIT

To obtain continuing pharmacy education (CE) credit for this program, **Safe Handling of Hazardous Drugs Video Training Program ACPE Program Number: 204-000-06-093-H04,** you must successfully pass the online test on the ASHP CE Testing Center at http://www.ashp.org/ce/homepage.cfm. If you score 70% or higher, you will be able to immediately print your CE statement. You will have two opportunities to pass the CE test. Also you can start, save, and exit the test at any time and be able to return to submit your final answers.

Use your 8-digit ASHP Member/Customer ID to log on (be sure to include any leading zeroes). Your member/Customer ID can be found on your membership card or on the mailing label of your copy of *AJHP*. To log on, click on "Enter the CE Testing Center" and type your ID number and password. Follow the instructions (below) to pay the CE Exam Processing Fee and also to select the CE test for **Safe Handling of Hazardous Drugs Video Training Program.**

If you are not an ASHP member or don't have a customer ID, you have two options to get one:

- Click on the link to obtain an ASHP Customer ID at http://www.ashp.org/ce/homepage.cfm
- Make a purchase at our shopping cart https://shop.ashp.org/timssnet/products/tnt_showprdsplash.cfm. An ASHP Customer ID and password would automatically be created for you.

Cannot remember your password? Click on the "forgot password" link at http://www.ashp.org/ce/homepage.cfm

Program Title: Safe Handling of Hazardous Drugs Video Training Program
ACPE Program # 204-000-06-093-H04
CE credit: 6 hours (0.6 CEU)

CE Exam Processing Fee: There is a nominal fee to access the test on the CE testing center. The fee for ASHP members is $20.95, and for non-ASHP members it is $30.95.

Go the ASHP Shopping Cart (http://shop.ashp. org/timssnet/products/tnt_showprdsplash.cfm) and select "Continuing Education." Click on "Add to Cart" icon and checkout. You can access the CE Testing Center immediately after your purchase to begin to take the CE test.

Questions: Call ASHP Customer Service Center toll free at (866) 279-0681.

 The American Society of Health-System Pharmacists is accredited by the Accreditation Council for Pharmacy Education as a provider for continuing pharmacy education.

Introduction

Concern regarding the safety of workers handling cytotoxic and hazardous drugs initially surfaced in the 1970s when reports of second cancers in patients treated with these agents were coupled with the discovery of mutagenic substances in the urine of nurses who handled these drugs and cared for treated patients.[1-3] The non-specific nature of the cytotoxic action of these drugs renders all cells at risk of DNA damage. This damage may be repaired by normal cell mechanisms or it may cause cell death or cell mutation, possibly leading to cancer.[4] Exposure to these drugs in the workplace has been associated with acute and long-term reactions. Anecdotal reports in the literature range from malaise and flu-like symptoms, to hair loss, nail damage, and mucosal sores.[5-8] Reproductive studies on health care workers have shown an increase in fetal abnormality, fetal loss, and fertility impairment resulting from occupational exposure to these potent drugs.[9-12] Increased incidence of cancers for these exposed groups has been investigated with varying success.[13,14] The small number of individuals available for study presents a dilemma for the statistician.

To reduce the amount of exposure to workers, numerous groups promulgated guidelines to improve the methods by which these drugs were handled in the workplace. The Occupational Safety and Health Administration (OSHA), the National Institutes of Health (NIH), the Oncology Nursing Society (ONS), and the American Society of Health-System Pharmacists (ASHP) developed recommendations for the safe handling of these agents in numerous health-care settings (refer to http://www.ashp.org/bestpractices/drugdistribution/Prep_Gdl_HazDrugs.pdf).[15-19] While the guidelines differ in some respects, the general principles and goals are very similar: establish and maintain stringent work practices within a framework of engineering controls and personal protective equipment to reduce the amount of drug released into the environment during manipulation. Subsequently, this reduction in available drug will reduce the potential exposure to personnel as well.

Despite implementation of these guidelines in the mid-1980s, continued research of areas where cytotoxics are manipulated shows both environmental contamination and worker contamination. Numerous studies report contamination on drug vials, work surfaces, gloves, and final product that has been transferred to workers. Concentrations of these cytotoxic agents have also been measured in the urine of workers who directly and superficially handle these drugs.[20-31]

In 1999, a multi-center study[32] conducted in the United States and Canada documented surface contamination in both compounding and administration of hazardous drugs utilizing published safe-handling equipment, personal protection, and work practices. While no single method of measuring and monitoring contamination and exposure has been found to be uniformly acceptable or useful,[33] the numerous positive findings along with the documented surface contamination require a reevaluation of the recommendations for the safe handling of hazardous drugs.[34]

REFERENCES

1. Weisburger JH, Griwold DP, Prejean JD, et al. Tumor induction by cytostatics. The carcinogenic properties of some of the principal drugs used in clinical cancer chemotherapy; recent results. *Cancer Res.* 1975; 52:1–17.
2. Harris CC. The carcinogenicity of anticancer drugs: a hazard in man. *Cancer.* 1976; 37:1014–1023.
3. Falck K, Grohn P, Sorsa M, et al. Mutagenicity in urine of nurses handling cytostatic drugs. *Lancet.* 1979; 1:1250–1251.
4. Harris CC. Immunosuppressive anticancer drugs in man: their oncogenic potential. *Radiology.* 1975; 114:163–166.

5. Ladik CF, Stoehr GP, Maurer MA. Precautionary measures in the preparation of antineoplastics. *Am J Hosp Pharm.* 1980; 37:1184, 1186.

6. Crudi CB. A compounding dilemma: I've kept the drug sterile but have I contaminated myself? *NITA.* 1980; 3:77–78.

7. Crudi CB, Stephens BL, Maier P. Possible occupational hazards associated with the preparation/administration of antineoplastic agents. *NITA.* 1982; 5:264–266.

8. Reynolds RD, Ignoffo R, Lawrence J, et al. Adverse reactions to AMSA in medical personnel. *Cancer Treat Rep.* 1982; 66:1885.

9. Hemminki K, Kyyronen P, Lindholm ML. Spontaneous abortions and malformations in the offspring of nurses exposed to anaesthetic gases, cytostatic drugs, and other potential hazards, based on registered information of outcome. *J Epidemiol Community Health.* 1985; 39:141–147.

10. Selevan SG, Linbohm ML, Hornung RW, et al. A study of occupational exposure to antineoplastic drugs and fetal loss in nurses. *New Engl J Med.* 1985; 313 (19):1173–1178.

11. Valanis B, Vollmer W, Labuhn K, et al. Occupational exposure to antineoplastic agents and self-reported infertility among nurses and pharmacists. *J Occup Environ Med.* 1997; 39:574–580.

12. Valanis B, Vollmer WM, Steele P. Occupational exposures to antineoplastic agents: self-reported miscarriages and stillbirths among nurses and pharmacists. *J Occup Environ Med.* 1999; 41:632–638.

13. Skov T, Lynge E, Maarup B, et al. Risks for physicians handling antineoplastic drugs. *Lancet.* 1990; 2:1446. Letter.

14. Skov T, Maarup B, Olsen J, et al. Leukaemia and reproductive outcome among nurses handling antineoplastic drugs. *Br J Ind Med.* 1992; 49:855–861.

15. Controlling occupational exposure to hazardous drugs. In: OSHA Technical Manual (OSHA Instruction CPL 2-2.20B CH-4). Washington,

DC: Directorate of Technical Support, Occupational Safety and Health Administration; 1995:Chap 21.

16. OSHA Technical Manual, TED 1-0.15A, Section VI, Chapter 2, Jan 20, 1999 (http://www.osha.gov/dts/osta/otm/otm_vi/otm_vi_2.html#2)

17. National Institutes of Health. Recommendations for the safe handling of cytotoxic drugs; 1992. Available at http://www. nih.gov/od/ors/ds/pubs/cyto/index.htm.

18. Polovich M, White J, Kelleher L. Chemotherapy and Biotherapy Guidelines and Recommendations for Practice. 2nd ed. Pittsburgh, PA: Oncology Nursing Society; 2005.

19. ASHP guidelines on handling hazardous drugs. *Am J Health-Syst Pharm*. In press. Refer to http://www.ashp.org/bestpractices/drugdistribution/Prep_Gdl_HazDrugs.pdf.

20. Ensslin AS, Pethran A, Schierl R, et al. Urinary platinum in hospital personnel occupationally exposed to platinum-containing antineoplastic drugs. *Int Arch Occup Environ Health*. 1994; 65:339–342.

21. Ensslin AS, Huber R, Pethran A, et al. Biological monitoring of hospital pharmacy personnel occupationally exposed to cytostatic drugs: urinary excretion and cytogenetics studies. *Int Arch Occup Environ Health*. 1997; 70:205–208.

22. Ensslin AS, Stoll Y, Pethran A, et al. Biological monitoring of cyclophosphamide and ifosfamide in urine of hospital personnel occupationally exposed to cytostatic drugs. *J Occup Environ Med*. 1994; 51:229–233.

23. Sessink PJM, Boer KA, Scheefhals APH, et al. Occupational exposure to antineoplastic agents at several departments in a hospital: Environmental contamination and excretion of cyclophosphamide and ifosfamide in urine of exposed workers. *Int Arch Occup Environ Health*. 1992; 64:105–112.

24. Sessink PJM, Van de Kerkhof MCA, Anzion RB, et al. Environmental contamination and assessment of exposure to antineoplastic agents by determination of cyclophosphamide

in urine of exposed pharmacy technicians: Is skin absorption an important exposure route? *Arch Environ Health*. 1994; 49:165–169.

25. Sessink PJM, Wittenhorst BCJ, Anzion RBM, et al. Exposure of pharmacy technicians to antineoplastic agents: reevaluation after additional protective measures. *Arch Environ Health*. 1997; 52:240–244.

26. Kiffmeyer TK, Ing KG, Schoppe G. External contamination of cytotoxic drug packing: safe handling and cleaning procedures. *J Onc Pharm Practice*. 2000; 6:13.

27. Minoia C, Turci R, Sottani C, et al. Application of high performance liquid chromatography/ tandem mass spectrometry in the environmental and biological monitoring of health care personnel occupationally exposed to cyclophosphamide and ifosfamide. *Rapid Commun Mass Spectrom*. 1998; 12:1485–1493.

28. Rubino FM, Floridia L, Pietropaolo AM, et al. Measurement of surface contamination by certain antineoplastic drugs using high-performance liquid chromatography: applications in occupational hygiene investigations in hospital environments. *Med Lav*. 1999; 90:572–583.

29. DeMeo MP, Merono S, DeBaille AD, et al. Monitoring exposure of hospital personnel handling cytostatic drugs and contaminated materials. *Int Arch Occup Environ Health*. 1995; 66:363–368.

30. Wick C, Slawson MH, Jorgenson JA, et al. Using a closed-system protective device to reduce personnel exposure to antineoplastic agents. *Am J Health-Syst Pharm*. 2003; 60:2314-2320.

31. Connor TH, Sessink PJM, Harrison BR, et al. Surface contamination of chemotherapy drug vials and evaluation of new vial-cleaning techniques: results of three studies. *Am J Health-Syst Pharm*. 2005; 62:475-484.

32. Connor TH, Anderson RW, Sessink PJM, et al. Surface contamination with antineoplastic agents in six cancer treatment centers in the United Sates and Canada. *Am J Health-Syst Pharm*. 1999; 56:1427–1432.

33. Baker ES, Connor TH. Monitoring occupational exposure to cancer chemotherapy drugs. *Am J Health-Syst Pharm.* 1996; 53:2713–2723.

34. Harrison BR. Exposure to hazardous drugs: time to reevaluate your program? [Editorial] *Am J Health-Syst Pharm.* 1999; 56:1403.

How to Use This Program

This program is designed so you can work at your own pace. You do not have to complete the exercises while viewing the video/DVD, but rather familiarize yourself with the content, then return, at a later time, to complete each exercise. Where relevant, you are given a list of supplies you will need to complete the exercises. It is important to complete as many of these exercises as you have been given in both the video/DVD and the workbook. The workbook also contains a glossary of terms with which you should become familiar. **Note:** *This program is not intended to replace or demonstrate best hands-on practices but rather provide an overview of the safe handling of cytotoxic and hazardous drugs and a foundation for best practices.*

You will notice that icons have been used to separate each section of the video/DVD. These icons will help you recognize which topic you were on when you paused the video/DVD.

You should work through the entire program first before reviewing any sections out of sequence. The self-assessment questions within each section are written to test your mastery of the subject. Please complete each one and record your answers in this workbook.

You are now invited to begin. Good luck and enjoy the program!

*We would like to thank the following companies for
their unrestricted educational support of this program.*

Baxa Corporation

Clinical IQ, LLC

Controlled Environment Consulting, Inc.

Lab Safety Corporation

Micro-Clean, Inc

Tyco Kendall-LTP

What Are Hazardous Drugs?

In Chapter 1, you will examine the definition of hazardous drugs, the criteria for determining which drugs are hazardous, and the potential health risks involved when handling these drugs.

OBJECTIVES

Upon completion of this chapter, you will be able to:

1. Define hazardous drugs.
2. Identify hazardous-drug criteria.
3. Describe the potential health risks of handling hazardous drugs.

DISCUSSION POINTS

Hazardous Drugs: Definition and Criteria

Hazardous drugs are drugs that pose a potential health risk to workers who may be exposed to them during receipt, transport, preparation, administration, or disposal. Such drugs require special handling because of their inherent toxicities. Although many hazardous drugs are cytotoxic, antineoplastic (chemotherapeutic) drugs, antiviral drugs, immunosuppressants, bioengineered drugs, and other types of drugs also may be hazardous The term *hazardous drugs* includes any drug that presents an occupational risk.

Drugs have a successful history of use in treating illnesses and injuries, and they are responsible for many of our medical advances over the past century. However, virtually all drugs have side effects. As these drugs are released into the environment during routine handling, workers and others in a contaminated area are at risk of suffering these effects. In addition, exposure to even very small amounts of certain drugs may be hazardous for workers.

The term *hazardous drug* was first used by the American Society of Health-System Pharmacists (ASHP) and is currently used by the Occupational Safety and Health Administration (OSHA). The 1990 "ASHP Technical Assistance Bulletin on Handling Cytotoxic and Hazardous Drugs"[1] proposed criteria to determine which drugs should be considered hazardous and handled within an established safety program. Drugs are classified as hazardous when studies in animals or humans indicate that exposure to them could cause cancer, developmental or reproductive toxicity, or harm to organs at low doses. OSHA adopted these criteria in their 1995 guidelines and posted them to their Web site in 1999.[2,3]

The 1990 ASHP definition of hazardous drugs was revised in 2004 by the National Institute for Occupational Safety and Health (NIOSH) Working

Group on Hazardous Drugs for the NIOSH Alert on hazardous drugs.[4,†] Drugs considered hazardous include those that exhibit one or more of the following six characteristics in humans or animals:

1. Carcinogenicity—causes cancer.
2. Teratogenicity—damages the developing fetus.
3. Reproductive toxicity—impairs fertility.
4. Organ toxicity at low doses.
5. Genotoxicity—damages DNA.
6. Structure and toxicity profiles of new drugs that mimic those of existing drugs that are hazardous by the above criteria.

Table 1-1 provides a sample list of hazardous drugs.[4,†]

The National Toxicology Program[5] and the International Agency for Research on Cancer[6] classify drugs according to carcinogenicity. Many antineoplastic drugs and immunosuppressants are included in their lists of known or suspected human carcinogens.

Many hazardous drugs used to treat cancer work by binding to or damaging DNA (for example, alkylating agents). Other antineoplastic drugs, some antivirals, antibiotics, and bioengineered drugs interfere with cell growth or proliferation, or with DNA synthesis. In some cases, the nonselective actions of these drugs disrupt the growth and function of both healthy and diseased cells, resulting in toxic side effects for treated patients. These nonselective actions also can cause adverse effects in health care workers who are inadvertently exposed to the drugs.

Concerns about occupational exposure to hazardous drugs first appeared in the 1970s. As the use and number of these potent drugs increase, so do opportunities for hazardous exposures among health care workers.

◀ **Key Idea** ▶

The term *hazardous drug* includes drugs that present an occupational risk.

---

†See the NIOSH Web site for updates to definition and Table 1-1.

Table 1-1
Sample List of Drugs that Should Be Handled as Hazardous[*,†]

Drug	Source	AHFS Pharmacologic–Therapeutic Classification
Aldesleukin	4, 5	10:00 Antineoplastic agents
Alemtuzumab	1, 3, 4, 5	10:00 Antineoplastic agents
Alitretinoin	3, 4, 5	84:36 Miscellaneous skin and mucous membrane agents (Retinoid)
Altretamine	1, 2, 3, 4, 5	Not in AHFS (Antineoplastic agent)
Amsacrine	3, 5	Not in AHFS (Antineoplastic agent)
Anastrozole	1, 5	10:00 Antineoplastic agents
Arsenic trioxide	1, 2, 3, 4, 5	10:00 Antineoplastic agents
Asparaginase	1, 2, 3, 4, 5	10:00 Antineoplastic agents
Azacitidine	3, 5	Not in AHFS (antineoplastic agent)
Azathioprine	2, 3, 5	92:00 Unclassified therapeutic agents (immunosuppressant)
Bexarotene	2, 3, 4, 5	10:00 Antineoplastic agents
Bicalutamide	1, 5	10:00 Antineoplastic agents
Bleomycin	1, 2, 3, 4, 5	10:00 Antineoplastic agents
Busulfan	1, 2, 3, 4, 5	10:00 Antineoplastic agents
Capecitabine	1, 2, 3, 4, 5	10:00 Antineoplastic agents
Carboplatin	1, 2, 3, 4, 5	10:00 Antineoplastic agents
Carmustine	1, 2, 3, 4, 5	10:00 Antineoplastic agents
Cetrorelix acetate	5	92:00 Unclassified therapeutic agents (GnRH antagonist)
Chlorambucil	1, 2, 3, 4, 5	10:00 Antineoplastic agents
Chloramphenicol	1, 5	8:12 Antibiotics
Choriogonadotropin alfa	5	68:18 Gonadotropins
Cidofovir	3, 5	8:18 Antivirals
Cisplatin	1, 2, 3, 4, 5	10:00 Antineoplastic agents

(See footnotes at end of table. Table continued)

Table 1-1 *(continued)*
Sample List of Drugs that Should Be Handled as Hazardous*,†

Drug	Source	AHFS Pharmacologic–Therapeutic Classification
Cladribine	1, 2, 3, 4, 5	10:00 Antineoplastic agents
Colchicine	5	92:00 Unclassified therapeutic agents (mitotic inhibitor)
Cyclophosphamide	1, 2, 3, 4, 5	10:00 Antineoplastic agents
Cytarabine	1, 2, 3, 4, 5	10:00 Antineoplastic agents
Cyclosporine	1	92:00 Immunosuppressive agents
Dacarbazine	1, 2, 3, 4, 5	10:00 Antineoplastic agents
Dactinomycin	1, 2, 3, 4, 5	10:00 Antineoplastic agents
Daunorubicin HCl	1, 2, 3, 4, 5	10:00 Antineoplastic agents
Denileukin	3, 4, 5	10:00 Antineoplastic agents
Dienestrol	5	68:16.04 Estrogens
Diethylstilbestrol	5	Not in AHFS (nonsteroidal synthetic estrogen)
Dinoprostone	5	76:00 Oxytocics
Docetaxel	1, 2, 3, 4, 5	10:00 Antineoplastic agents
Doxorubicin	1, 2, 3, 4, 5	10:00 Antineoplastic agents
Dutasteride	5	92:00 Unclassifed therapeutic agents (5-alpha reductase inhibitor)
Epirubicin	1, 2, 3, 4, 5	10:00 Antineoplastic agents
Ergonovine/methylergonovine	5	76:00 Oxytocics
Estradiol	1, 5	68:16.04 Estrogens
Estramustine phosphate sodium	1, 2, 3, 4, 5	10:00 Antineoplastic agents
Estrogen-progestin combinations	5	68:12 Contraceptives
Estrogens, conjugated	5	68:16.04 Estrogens
Estrogens, esterified	5	68:16.04 Estrogens
Estrone	5	68:16.04 Estrogens

(See footnotes at end of table. Table continued)

Table 1-1 *(continued)*
Sample List of Drugs that Should Be Handled as Hazardous*,†

Drug	Source	AHFS Pharmacologic–Therapeutic Classification
Estropipate	5	68:16.04 Estrogens
Etoposide	1, 2, 3, 4, 5	10:00 Antineoplastic agents
Exemestane	1, 5	10:00 Antineoplastic agents
Finasteride	1, 3, 5	92:00 Unclassified therapeutic Agents (5-alpha reductase inhibitor)
Floxuridine	1, 2, 3, 4, 5	10:00 Antineoplastic agents
Fludarabine	1, 2, 3, 4, 5	10:00 Antineoplastic agents
Fluorouracil	1, 2, 3, 4, 5	10:00 Antineoplastic agents
Fluoxymesterone	5	68:08 Androgens
Flutamide	1, 2, 5	10:00 Antineoplastic agents
Fulvestrant	5	10:00 Antineoplastic agents
Ganciclovir	1, 2, 3, 4, 5	8:18 Antiviral
Ganirelix acetate	5	92:00 Unclassified therapeutic agents (GnRH antagonist)
Gemcitabine	1, 2, 3, 4, 5	10:00 Antineoplastic agents
Gemtuzumab ozogamicin	1, 3, 4, 5	10:00 Antineoplastic agents
Gonadotropin, chorionic	5	68:18 Gonadotropins
Goserelin	1, 2, 5	10:00 Antineoplastic agents
Hydroxyurea	1, 2, 3, 4, 5	10:00 Antineoplastic agents
Ibritumomab tiuxetan	3	10:00 Antineoplastic agents
Idarubicin	1, 2, 3, 4, 5	Not in AHFS (antineoplastic agent)
Ifosfamide	1, 2, 3, 4, 5	10:00 Antineoplastic agents
Imatinib mesylate	1, 3, 4, 5	10:00 Antineoplastic agents
Interferon alfa-2a	1, 2, 4, 5	10:00 Antineoplastic agents
Interferon alfa-2b	1, 2, 4, 5	10:00 Antineoplastic agents

(See footnotes at end of table. Table continued)

Table 1-1 (continued)
Sample List of Drugs that Should Be Handled as Hazardous*,†

Drug	Source	AHFS Pharmacologic–Therapeutic Classification
Interferon alfa-n1	1, 5	10:00 Antineoplastic agents
Interferon alfa-n3	1, 5	10:00 Antineoplastic agents
Irinotecan HCl	1, 2, 3, 4, 5	10:00 Antineoplastic agents
Leflunomide	3, 5	92:00 Unclassified therapeutic agents (antineoplastic agent)
Letrozole	1, 5	10:00 Antineoplastic agents
Leuprolide acetate	1, 2, 5	10:00 Antineoplastic agents
Lomustine	1, 2, 3, 4, 5	10:00 Antineoplastic agents
Mechlorethamine	1, 2, 3, 4, 5	10:00 Antineoplastic agents
Megestrol	1, 5	10:00 Antineoplastic agents
Melphalan	1, 2, 3, 4, 5	10:00 Antineoplastic agents
Menotropins	5	68:18 Gonadotropins
Mercaptopurine	1, 2, 3, 4, 5	10:00 Antineoplastic agents
Methotrexate	1, 2, 3, 4, 5	10:00 Antineoplastic agents
Methyltestosterone	5	68:08 Androgens
Mifepristone	5	76:00 Oxytocics
Mitomycin	1, 2, 3, 4, 5	10:00 Antineoplastic agents
Mitotane	1, 4, 5	10:00 Antineoplastic agents
Mitoxantrone HCl	1, 2, 3, 4, 5	10:00 Antineoplastic agents
Mycophenolate mofetil	1, 3, 5	92:00 Immunosuppressive agents
Nafarelin	5	68:18 Gonadotropins
Nilutamide	1, 5	10:00 Antineoplastic agents
Oxaliplatin	1, 3, 4, 5	10:00 Antineoplastic agents
Oxytocin	5	76:00 Oxytocics
Paclitaxel	1, 2, 3, 4, 5	10:00 Antineoplastic agents

(See footnotes at end of table. Table continued)

Table 1-1 *(continued)*
Sample List of Drugs that Should Be Handled as Hazardous*,†

Drug	Source	AHFS Pharmacologic–Therapeutic Classification
Pegaspargase	1, 2, 3, 4, 5	10:00 Antineoplastic agents
Pentamidine isethionate	1, 2, 3, 5	8:40 Miscellaneous anti-infectives
Pentostatin	1, 2, 3, 4, 5	10:00 Antineoplastic agents
Perphosphamide	3, 5	Not in AHFS (antineoplastic agent)
Pipobroman	3, 5	Not in AHFS (antineoplastic agent)
Piritrexim isethionate	3, 5	Not in AHFS (antineoplastic agent)
Plicamycin	1, 2, 3, 5	Not in AHFS (antineoplastic agent)
Podofilox	5	84:36 Miscellaneous skin and mucous membrane agents (mitotic inhibitor)
Podophyllum resin	5	84:36 Miscellaneous skin and mucous membrane agents (mitotic inhibitor)
Prednimustine	3, 5	Not in AHFS (antineoplastic agent)
Procarbazine	1, 2, 3, 4, 5	10:00 Antineoplastic agents
Progesterone	5	68:32 Progestins
Progestins	5	68:12 Contraceptives
Raloxifene	5	68:16.12 Estrogen agonists-antagonists
Raltitrexed	5	Not in AHFS (antineoplastic agent)
Ribavirin	1, 2, 5	8:18 Antiviral
Streptozocin	1, 2, 3, 4, 5	10:00 Antineoplastic agents
Tacrolimus	1, 5	92:00 Unclassified therapeutic agents (immunosuppressant)
Tamoxifen	1, 2, 5	10:00 Antineoplastic agents
Temozolomide	3, 4, 5	10:00 Antineoplastic agents
Teniposide	1, 2, 3, 4, 5	10:00 Antineoplastic agents
Testolactone	5	10:00 Antineoplastic agents
Testosterone	5	68:08 Androgens

(See footnotes at end of table. Table continued)

Table 1-1 *(continued)*

Sample List of Drugs that Should Be Handled as Hazardous*,†

Drug	Source	AHFS Pharmacologic–Therapeutic Classification
Thalidomide	1, 3, 5	92:00 Unclassified therapeutic agents (immunomodulator)
Thioguanine	1, 2, 3, 4, 5	10:00 Antineoplastic agents
Thiotepa	1, 2, 3, 4, 5	10:00 Antineoplastic agents
Topotecan	1, 2, 3, 4, 5	10:00 Antineoplastic agents
Toremifene citrate	1, 5	10:00 Antineoplastic agents
Tositumomab	3, 5	Not in AHFS (antineoplastic agent)
Tretinoin	1, 2, 3, 5	84:16 Cell stimulants and proliferants (retinoid)
Trifluridine	1, 2, 5	52:04.06 antivirals
Trimetrexate glucuronate	5	8:40 Miscellaneous anti-infectives (folate antagonist)
Triptorelin	5	10:00 Antineoplastic agents
Uracil mustard	3, 5	Not in AHFS (antineoplastic agent)
Valganciclovir	1, 3, 5	8:18 Antiviral
Valrubicin	1, 2, 3, 5	10:00 Antineoplastic agents
Vidarabine	1, 2, 5	52:04.06 Antivirals
Vinblastine sulfate	1, 2, 3, 4, 5	10:00 Antineoplastic agents
Vincristine sulfate	1, 2, 3, 4, 5	10:00 Antineoplastic agents
Vindesine	1, 5	Not in AHFS (antineoplastic agent)
Vinorelbine tartrate	1, 2, 3, 4, 5	10:00 Antineoplastic agents
Zidovudine	1, 2, 5	8:18:08 Antiretroviral agents

*These lists of hazardous drugs were used with the permission of the institutions that provided them and were adapted for use by NIOSH. The sample lists are intended to guide health care providers in diverse practice settings and should not be construed as complete representations of all of the hazardous drugs used at the referenced institutions. Some drugs de ned as hazardous may not pose a significant risk of direct occupational exposure because of their dosage formulation (for example, intact medications such as coated tablets or capsules that are administered to patients without modifying the formulation). However, they may pose a risk if solid drug formulations are altered outside a ventilated cabinet (for example, if tablets are crushed or dissolved, or if capsules are pierced or opened).

†See the NIOSH Web site for updates to definition and Table 1-1.

(See footnotes at end of table. Table continued)

Table 1-1 *(continued)*
Sample List of Drugs that Should Be Handled as Hazardous*,†

[1]The NIH Clinical Center, Bethesda, MD (Revised 8/2002).

[2]The Johns Hopkins Hospital, Baltimore, MD (Revised 9/2002).

[3]The Northside Hospital, Atlanta, GA (Revised 8/2002).

[4]The University of Michigan Hospitals and Health Centers, Ann Arbor, MI (Revised 2/2003).

[5]This sample listing of hazardous drugs was compiled by the Pharmaceutical Research and Manufacturers of America (PhRMA) using information from the AHFS DI monographs published by ASHP in selected AHFS Pharmacologic–Therapeutic Classification categories [ASHP/AHFS DI 2003] and applying the definition for hazardous drugs. The list also includes drugs from other sources that satisfy the definition for hazardous drugs [PDR 2004; Sweetman 2002; Shepard 2001; Schardein 2000; REPROTOX 2003]. Newly approved drugs that have structures or toxicological profiles that mimic the drugs on this list should also be included. This list was revised in June 2004. [ASHP/AHFS DI 2003] and applying the definition for hazardous drugs. The list also includes drugs from other sources that satisfy the definition for hazardous drugs [PDR 2004; Sweetman 2002; Shepard 2001; Schardein 2000; REPROTOX 2003]. Newly approved drugs that have structures or toxicological profiles that mimic the drugs on this list should also be included. This list was revised in June 2004.

The Federal Hazard Communication Standards (HCS)

The federal Hazard Communication Standard ([HCS] CFR 1910.1200)[7,8] defines a chemical as hazardous if it poses a physical or a health risk. It further defines a chemical as a health hazard when there is statistically significant evidence based on at least one study conducted in accordance with established scientific principles that acute or chronic health effects may occur in exposed employees. The HCS notes that the term *health hazard* includes chemicals that are carcinogens, toxic or highly toxic agents, reproductive toxins, irritants, corrosives, sensitizers, and agents that produce target organ effects.

SUMMARY

Clearly defining terms such as hazardous drugs helps protect health care workers from occupational exposure to potentially harmful medications. A hazardous drug is currently defined by ASHP and NIOSH as a drug that poses a risk to a health care worker by virtue of its carcinogenic, mutagenic, teratogenic, or reproductive-toxicity potential. Although drugs categorized as hazardous generally include those used for the chemotherapy of cancer, many other drugs also are included.

REFERENCES

1. ASHP guidelines on handling hazardous drugs. *Am J Health-Syst Pharm*. In press. Refer to http://www.ashp.org/bestpractices/ drugdistribution/Prep_Gdl_HazDrugs.pdf.

2. Controlling occupational exposure to hazardous drugs. In: OSHA Technical Manual (OSHA Instruction CPL 2-2.20B CH-4). Washington, DC: Directorate of Technical Support, Occupational Safety and Health Administration; 1995:Chap 21.

3. Controlling occupational exposure to hazardous drugs. In: OSHA Technical Manual, TED 1-0.15A. Section VI: Chapter 2. January 20, 1999. Available at: http://www.osha.gov/dts/ osta/otm/otm_vi/otm_vi_2.html#2.

4. NIOSH Alert: Preventing Occupational Exposures to Antineoplastic and Other Hazardous Drugs in Healthcare Settings. Atlanta, GA: Centers for Disease Control and Prevention, National Institute for Occupational Safety and Health; 2004. DHHS (NIOSH) publication 2004-165. Available at: http://www.cdc.gov/ niosh/docs/2004-165/.

5. U.S. Department of Health and Human Services, National Toxicology Program. Report on Carcinogens. 11th ed. Available at: http:// ehis.niehs.nih.gov/roc/toc9.html. Accessed September 26, 2005.

6. International Agency for Research on Cancer. IARC monographs on the evaluation of carcinogenic risks to humans. 2005. Available at: http://www-cie.iarc.fr/. Accessed September 26, 2005.

7. Hazard Communication Standard. 29 CFR Part 1910.1200. Available at: http://www. osha.gov/pls/oshaweb/owadisp.show_ document?p_table=STANDARDS&p_id=10099. Accessed September 26, 2005.

8. Occupational Safety and Health Administration. Hazard Communication Standard. Final Rules. *Fed Regist*. 1987; 52:31852–31886.

EXERCISE

Generate a list of hazardous drugs specific to your facility. If a list is already in place, compare it to the list in Table 1-1 (the NIOSH Alert).[4] A practice-specific list of hazardous drugs should be comprehensive, including all hazardous medications routinely used or very likely to be used by your facility. Make sure that all personnel can access this list.

SELF-ASSESSMENT

1. Which organization first used the term *hazardous drug*?

   A. ASHP.
   B. OSHA.
   C. NIOSH.
   D. Oncology Nursing Society (ONS).

2. Which term defines hazardous drugs as damaging the developing fetus?

   A. Carcinogenicity.
   B. Teratogenicity.
   C. Genotoxicity.
   D. Reproductive toxicity.

3. As the use and number of these potent drugs increase, so do opportunities for hazardous exposures among health care workers.

   A. True.
   B. False.

4. Which term is most preferred when discussing drugs that may put workers exposed to them at risk?

    A. Cytotoxic.
    B. Chemotherapy.
    C. Antineoplastic.
    D. Hazardous.

5. Which organization classifies drugs according to carcinogenicity?

    A. ASHP.
    B. NIOSH.
    C. International Agency for Research on Cancer (IARC).
    D. National Institutes of Health (NIH).

Return to video ▶

ASHP and Other Guidelines

In Chapter 2, you will examine the various guidelines used to handle hazardous drugs.

OBJECTIVES

Upon completion of this chapter, you will be able to:

1. Summarize the latest American Society of Health-System Pharmacists (ASHP) guidelines on handling hazardous drugs.
2. Summarize the goals of the National Institute for Occupational Safety and Health (NIOSH) and the National Occupational Research Agenda (NORA) as they pertain to the safe handling of hazardous drugs.
3. Identify Occupational Safety and Health Administration (OSHA) guidelines on handling hazardous drugs.
4. Explain the relationship of the U.S. Environmental Protection Agency (EPA) to the management of hazardous drugs.

DISCUSSION POINTS

ASHP Guidelines

In 1990, ASHP issued the revised "ASHP Technical Assistance Bulletin on Handling Cytotoxic and Hazardous Drugs" (TAB).[1] Information and recommendations contained in that document were current to June 1988. Continuing reports of workplace contamination and concerns for the safety of health care workers prompted OSHA to issue new guidelines on controlling occupational exposure to hazardous drugs in 1995.[2]

In 2004, NIOSH issued the *NIOSH Alert: Preventing Occupational Exposures to Antineoplastic and Other Hazardous Drugs in Healthcare Settings.*[3] The Oncology Nursing Society (ONS) issued *Chemotherapy and Biotherapy Guidelines and Recommendation for Practice* in 2001[4] and 2005[5] as well as *Safe Handling of Hazardous Drugs* in 2003.[6] The new ASHP guidelines on handling hazardous drugs[7] include information from these recommendations and are current to 2005.

The purpose of these new ASHP guidelines is to update the reader on new and continuing concerns for health care workers who handle hazardous drugs and to provide information on recommendations, including equipment, that have been developed since the publication of the previous TAB.[1] As studies show that contamination occurs in many settings, these guidelines should be implemented wherever hazardous drugs are stored, prepared, administered, and disposed of.

Comprehensive reviews of the literature covering anecdotal and case reports of surface contamination, worker contamination, and risk assessment are available in the OSHA guidelines and in the NIOSH Alert, as well as from individual authors.[2–4,8–10]

OSHA

There should be a plan in place at your health care facility for determining which drugs are considered hazardous using ASHP, NIOSH, and OSHA criteria. Pharmacists, health care practitioners, and occupational health and safety specialists should be involved in developing policies and practices for safe handling of hazardous drugs. The pharmacist should take the lead in developing policies and practices for the safe handling of hazardous drugs. Under OSHA's Hazard Communication Standard,[11,12] health care workers are entitled to obtain from their employer the material safety data sheet (MSDS) for any hazardous agent to which they might be exposed, including a drug intended for a patient.

OSHA has identified worker exposure to hazardous drugs as an increasingly serious health concern.[2] Manufacturing, receiving, preparation, administration, and disposal of hazardous drugs may expose hundreds of thousands of workers, principally in health care facilities and the pharmaceutical industry, to potentially significant workplace levels of these drugs. Antineoplastics, cytotoxics, anesthetic agents, antivirals, and others have been identified as hazardous. These hazardous drugs are capable of causing serious effects including cancer, organ toxicity, fertility problems, genetic damage, and birth defects.

NIOSH/NORA Group

In 2000, NIOSH, in conjunction with NORA, convened a group of individuals interested in occupational exposure to hazardous drugs. The resulting work group includes representation from government [OSHA, NIOSH, Food and Drug Administration (FDA)], industry, pharmaceutical manufacturing, academia, membership organizations (e.g., ASHP, the Joint Commission on Accreditation of Healthcare Organizations, ONS), and union leaders whose members handle hazardous drugs.

The goals of the working group were to assess existing information on occupational exposure, increase awareness of the risks to the affected

◀ **Key Idea** ▶

OHSA has identified worker exposure to hazardous drugs as an increasingly serious health concern.[2]

workers, and determine appropriate plans of action to reduce these risks. The purpose of the 2004 NIOSH Alert[3] is to inform health care workers of the continuing risk of exposure and to outline the responsibility of employers and health care workers related to safe handling.

The following are recommendations from the NIOSH Alert[3] for employers and health care workers:

Employer responsibilities:
- Develop a written policy for the medical surveillance of personnel handling hazardous drugs. This policy must address drug handling during pregnancy.
- Develop policies and procedures for the safe receipt, storage, transport, preparation, administration, and disposal of hazardous drugs.
- Identify those hazardous drugs used in the facility and determine methods for updating the list.
- Provide mandatory training for all employees based on their hazardous drug-handling tasks.
- Make guidance documents such as MSDSs available to health care workers who handle hazardous drugs.
- Provide and maintain appropriate ventilated cabinets designed to protect workers and others from exposure to hazardous drugs. Examples of such cabinets include biological safety cabinets (BSCs) (Class II or III) and containment isolators.
- Provide personal protective equipment (PPE) designated for the purpose of handling hazardous drugs.
- Require that all employees who handle hazardous drugs wear appropriate PPE.
- Develop a hazardous-drug spill management policy and procedure.
- Monitor compliance with safe-handling policies and procedures.

Health care worker responsibilities:
- Participate in training before handling hazardous drugs and update knowledge based on new information.

- Refer to guidance documents as necessary for information regarding hazardous drugs.
- Utilize appropriate ventilated cabinet when compounding drugs.
- Use recommended gloves, gowns, eye, face and respiratory protection.
- Wash hands after drug-handling activities and removal of PPE.
- Dispose of materials contaminated with hazardous drugs separately from other waste in designated containers.
- Clean up hazardous-drug spills immediately according to recommended procedures.
- Follow institutional procedures for reporting and following up on accidental exposure to hazardous drugs.

EPA

The U.S. EPA regulations under the Resource Conservation and Recovery Act (RCRA) require that hazardous waste be managed by following a strict set of regulatory requirements (40 CFR Parts 260–279). Disposal of hazardous materials and toxic chemicals continues to be a controversial issue, of which the disposal of hazardous drugs is but a small part.

The EPA currently issues permits for management of hazardous waste. Some contractors may purport to possess permits to handle these types of hazardous agents when, in fact, they do not meet the requirements or are only in the initial stages of obtaining permits. It is imperative that health care facilities verify the license or permit status of any contractor used to remove or dispose of infectious or hazardous waste.

Published EPA guidelines include the following:

- *Managing Hazardous Waste: A Guide for Small Businesses.* 2001.
- *RCRA Hazardous Waste Regulations.* 40 CFR Parts 260–279.

SUMMARY

OSHA, ASHP, ONS, and NIOSH all provide guidelines for the safe handling of hazardous drugs. Although adherence to these recommendations does not provide complete protection, it is believed that adherence will reduce health care workers' exposure. When exposure is reduced, the negative health effects also should be reduced. It is time for health care workers to take their own occupational safety as seriously as the safety of the patients under their care.

REFERENCES

1. ASHP technical assistance bulletin on handling cytotoxic and hazardous drugs. *Am J Hosp Pharm.* 1990; 47:1033–1049.
2. Controlling occupational exposure to hazardous drugs. In: OSHA Technical Manual (OSHA Instruction CPL 2-2.20B CH-4). Washington, DC: Directorate of Technical Support, Occupational Safety and Health Administration; 1995:Chap 21.
3. NIOSH Alert: Preventing Occupational Exposures to Antineoplastic and Other Hazardous Drugs in Healthcare Settings. Atlanta, GA: Centers for Disease Control and Prevention, National Institute for Occupational Safety and Health; 2004. DHHS (NIOSH) publication 2004-165.
4. Brown KA, Esper P, Kelleher LO, et al. Chemotherapy and Biotherapy Guidelines and Recommendations for Practice. Pittsburgh, PA: Oncology Nursing Society; 2001.
5. Polovich M, White J, Kelleher L. Chemotherapy and Biotherapy Guidelines and Recommendations for Practice. 2nd ed. Pittsburgh, PA: Oncology Nursing Society; 2005.
6. Polovich M, ed. Safe Handling of Hazardous Drugs. Pittsburgh, PA: Oncology Nursing Society; 2003.
7. American Society of Health-System Pharmacists. ASHP guidelines on handling hazardous drugs. *Am J Health-Syst Pharm.* In press. Refer

to http://www.ashp.org/bestpractices/drugdistribution/Prep_Gdl_HazDrugs.pdf.

8. Controlling occupational exposure to hazardous drugs. In: OSHA Technical Manual, TED 1-0.15A. Section VI: Chapter 2. January 20, 1999. Available at: http://www.osha.gov/dts/osta/otm/otm_vi/otm_vi_2.html#2.

9. Harrison BR. Risks of handling cytotoxic drugs. In: Perry MC, ed. The Chemotherapy Source Book. 3rd ed. Philadelphia, PA: Lippincott, Williams and Wilkins; 2001:566–582.

10. Sessink PJM, Bos RP. Drugs hazardous to healthcare workers: evaluation of methods for monitoring occupational exposure to cytostatic drugs. *Drug Saf.* 1999; 20:347–359.

11. Hazard Communication Standard. 29 CFR Part 1910.1200. Available at: http://www.osha.gov/pls/oshaweb/owadisp.show_document?p_table=STANDARDS&p_id=10099. Accessed September 26, 2005.

12. Occupational Safety and Health Administration. Hazard Communication Standard. Final Rules. *Fed Regist.* 1987; 52:31852–31886.

EXERCISE

Download a copy of the *ASHP Guidelines on Handling Hazardous Drugs* at: http://www.ashp.org/bestpractices/drugdistribution/Gdl_HazDrugs.pdf.

SELF-ASSESSMENT

1. Which statement best describes the purpose of the ASHP guidelines on handling hazardous drugs?

   A. To update the reader on new and continuing concerns for health care workers who handle hazardous drugs.

   B. To reevaluate previous versions of the guidelines for errors.

   C. To present standard operating procedures for the handling of hazardous drugs.

D. To provide continuing education through documentation regarding the handling of hazardous drugs.

2. So far, only ASHP and NIOSH have provided guidelines for the safe handling of hazardous drugs.

   A. True.
   B. False.

3. Special training is mandatory for all employees who handle hazardous drugs.

   A. True.
   B. False.

4. The pharmacist should take the lead in developing policies and practices for the safe handling of hazardous drugs.

   A. True.
   B. False.

5. Which governmental agency mandates the availability of MSDSs for any hazardous chemical or drug?

   A. OSHA.
   B. FDA.
   C. NIOSH.
   D. EPA.

Return to video ▶

Receipt, Storage, Labeling, and Transport

In Chapter 3, you will explore the various labeling and packaging guidelines that deal specifically with hazardous drugs.

OBJECTIVES

Upon completion of this chapter, you will be able to:

1. Receive and unpack drug shipments, including hazardous drugs.
2. Describe proper storage techniques for hazardous drugs.
3. Define labeling procedures for hazardous drugs.
4. Package hazardous-drug products for transport within a facility.

DISCUSSION POINTS

Receipt and Storage

The Hazard Communication Standard[1,2] applies to all workers, including those handling hazardous drugs at the manufacturer and distributor level. Appropriate controls should be in place to ensure safe distribution of these drugs.

Cartons of such drugs transported from the manufacturer or distributor should be labeled with an acceptable identifier to notify personnel receiving them to wear appropriate personal protective equipment (PPE) when opening the cartons. Sealing these drugs in plastic at the distributor level provides additional safety for workers who are required to unpack cartons.

Examination of such cartons for any outward sign of damage or breakage is an important first step in the receiving process. Policies and procedures must be in place for handling damaged cartons or containers of hazardous drugs. These may include returning the damaged goods to the distributor after applying appropriate containment techniques. Any handling of damaged hazardous drugs must be done using appropriate protective controls, including gloves and respiratory protection. Staff engaged in this practice must be fit-tested for the appropriate respirator, and respirators must be available at all times.[3]

Hazardous drugs should be separated from other drugs. Drug packages, bins, shelves, and all storage areas for hazardous drugs must bear distinctive labels identifying them as requiring special precautions. Segregation of hazardous-drug inventory improves control and reduces the number of staff members potentially exposed to the danger.

Hazardous drugs placed in inventory must be protected from potential breakage by storing in bins that have high fronts and on shelves that have guards to prevent accidental falling. The bins also must be the right size to properly contain all the stock. Care should be taken to separate inventory to reduce potential drug errors (e.g., pulling a look-a-like vial from an adjacent drug bin). As several studies have shown that contamination on the drug vial itself is a consideration, all staff members must wear double gloves when doing stocking, inventory control, or selecting drug packages for further handling.[4]

The following guidelines provided by the National Institute for Occupational Safety and Health (NIOSH) should be followed when receiving and storing hazardous drugs:

- Begin exposure control when hazardous drugs enter the facility. The most significant exposure risk during distribution and transport is from spills resulting from damaged containers.
- Prepare workers for the possibility that spills might occur while they are handling containers (even when packaging is intact during routine activities), and provide them with appropriate PPE.
- Make sure that drug cartons have labeling on the outside of containers that will be understood by all workers who will be separating hazardous from nonhazardous drugs.
- Wear two pairs of chemotherapy gloves, protective clothing, and eye protection when opening containers to unpack hazardous drugs. Such PPE protects workers and helps prevent contamination from spreading if damaged containers are found.
- Store hazardous drugs separately from other drugs, as recommended by the American Society of Health-System Pharmacists[5] and other chemical safety standards.
- Store and transport hazardous drugs in closed containers that minimize the risk of breakage.
- Make sure the storage area has sufficient general exhaust ventilation to dilute and remove any airborne contaminants.

Labeling

All hazardous drugs must be labeled in order to identify them for special handling. A label on the

◀ **Key Idea** ▶

Segregation of hazardous-drug inventory improves control and reduces the number of staff members potentially exposed to the danger.

◆ **Best Practice** ◆
Protect hazardous-drug inventory from potential breakage by storing in bins that have high fronts and on shelves that have guards.

drug container itself and on the outside of the bag used for transport should alert the handler that special precautions are required.

■ Labels should be specifically designed and should identify the preparation as hazardous.
■ Labels should state the storage requirements and beyond-use dating.
■ Other special labels also should be attached, where appropriate, to convey additional information or advice (e.g., do not administer intrathecally).
■ All safety/warning labels should be applied to both the immediate container and any outer safety packaging (e.g., transport bags containing final product).

Transporting from Pharmacy to Unit

All transport of hazardous-drug packages must be done in sealed containers to reduce contamination in the event that the package is accidentally dropped. Hazardous drugs need to be fully labeled and transported in secondary-closed containers to prevent exposure during impact or abusive handling. Staff transporting hazardous drugs need to be trained to recognize warning labels and damaged packaging, to control a spill site, and to report spills or overexposure. A spill kit must be available during transport.

The following are recommended guidelines:

■ Cartons of hazardous drugs that are received damaged should be examined, then opened, in an isolated area by an employee wearing approved double gloves, respirator, and other protective clothing.
■ Damaged containers and contaminated packaging materials should be contained, placed in puncture-resistant receptacles, and then returned to the manufacturer or distributor, if appropriate, or disposed of as hazardous waste.
■ Appropriate protective equipment, spill containment supplies, and waste-disposal materi-

---

◆ **Best Practice** ◆
Attach a warning label stating, for example,

"CAUTION: HAZARDOUS DRUG. HANDLE WITH GLOVES. DISPOSE OF PROPERLY."

als should be kept in the area where shipments are received.

■ Transport of hazardous drugs within a facility should be in sealed, primary-containment bags. All drugs should be labeled clearly. Spill kits must be readily available.

■ Methods that produce stress on contents, such as pneumatic tubes, should not be used to transport hazardous drugs.

SUMMARY

Many available guidelines address the safe handling of hazardous drugs. Proper receipt, storage, labeling, discarding, and transporting of hazardous drugs cannot be overlooked when considering worker safety. Workers at the receiving and transporting end are as much at risk as those who work directly with the hazardous drugs. Proper training of all workers who may be in contact with hazardous drugs is the most effective way to reduce the possibility of exposure.

REFERENCES

1. Hazard Communication Standard. 29 CFR Part 1910.1200. Available at: http://www. osha.gov/pls/oshaweb/owadisp.show_ document?p_table=STANDARDS&p_id=10099. Accessed September 26, 2005.

2. Occupational Safety and Health Administration. Hazard Communication Standard. Final Rules. *Fed Regist.* 1987; 52:31852–31886.

3. U.S. Department of Labor. Respiratory protection standard. 29 CFR Part 1910.134. Washington, DC: Occupational Safety and Health Administration; 1984.

4. ASHP guidelines on handling hazardous drugs. *Am J Health-Syst Pharm.* In press. Refer to http://www.ashp.org/bestpractices/ drugdistribution/Prep_Gdl_HazDrugs.pdf.

5. ASHP technical assistance bulletin on handling cytotoxic and hazardous drugs. *Am J Hosp Pharm.* 1990; 47:1033–1049.

EXERCISES

1. Examine your departmental policies and procedures for receipt, storage, labeling, and transporting of hazardous drugs. Do they meet the recommendations outlined in this chapter? Describe which steps (if any) are missing. What additional precautions does your facility take beyond those outlined to ensure personnel safety?

2. List the requirements that your facility has for the delivery of hazardous drugs from the distributor or manufacturer. Are the containers of hazardous drugs identified on the outside for the receiving staff's safety? Does the distributor repackage hazardous drugs in sealed plastic to ensure containment of any broken or damaged product?

SELF-ASSESSMENT

1. Which statement about transporting of hazardous drugs is TRUE?

   A. Transporting hazardous-drug packages must be in sealed containers.
   B. Secondary-closed containers are not needed for transporting hazardous drugs.
   C. Damaged cartons that are received should be destroyed immediately.
   D. Protective equipment and waste-disposal materials should be kept in an area separate from that where shipments are received.

2. Which statement BEST describes the proper storage of hazardous drugs?

   A. Hazardous drugs may be stored with other drugs.
   B. Segregation of hazardous-drug inventory decreases control.
   C. Once hazardous drugs are stored, staff members only need to wear gloves when manipulating them.

D. Hazardous-drug packages, bins, shelves and all storage areas must bear distinctive labels.

3. Hazardous-drug safety labels need only appear on the outside of packaging.

   A. True.
   B. False.

4. The Hazard Communication Standard applies only to pharmacy workers.

   A. True.
   B. False.

5. Staff who receive shipping cartons of hazardous drugs must be fully trained in the use of PPE, including respirators.

   A. True.
   B. False.

Return to video ▶

Risk Assessment, Controls, and Medical Surveillance

In Chapter 4, you will review the elements of risk assessment and medical surveillance.

OBJECTIVES

Upon completion of this chapter, you will be able to:

1. Define the elements of a safety program.
2. Explain the risks involved in the exposure to hazardous drugs, including the possible relationship between environmental contamination and drug uptake into the body.
3. Describe environmental and ventilation controls used to reduce exposure to hazardous drugs.
4. Define medical surveillance.

DISCUSSION POINTS

A comprehensive safety program must be developed that deals with all aspects of the safe handling of hazardous drugs. This program must be a collaborative effort with input from all affected departments, such as pharmacy, nursing, medical staff, housekeeping, transportation, maintenance, employee health, risk management, industrial hygiene, clinical laboratories, and safety officers.[1] Only authorized and adequately trained personnel should receive, prepare, transport, or administer hazardous drugs.

Risk Assessment

Risk assessment is a process by which we evaluate the potential for adverse health or environmental effects either from naturally occurring sources or from external sources like hazardous drugs. A thorough risk assessment typically includes an estimate of the probability of harm and a clear description of the various assumptions and uncertainties that contribute to risk. Unfortunately, a formal risk assessment of a work site is not always available to practitioners. However, an alternative is a performance-based, observational approach. Given the results of the numerous contamination studies, observation of current work practices will serve as an initial assessment of appropriate and inappropriate practices. Comparing a work site with one reported in the literature will provide an initial assessment of possible contamination and subsequent risk. For example, surface contamination with cyclophosphamide has been associated with the presence of cyclophosphamide in the urine.[2-4] Vandenbroucke and Robays[2] found that cyclophosphamide was excreted in the urine of four of six persons engaged in processing hazardous drugs using standard preparation techniques.

Wick et al[3] reported cyclophosphamide in 14 of 39 urine samples obtained from five pharmacy personnel (three of the five were positive for

> ◀ **Key Idea** ▶
>
> **Risk assessment is a process by which we evaluate the potential for adverse health or environmental effects either from naturally occurring sources or from external sources like hazardous drugs.**

cyclophosphamide) preparing hazardous drugs using standard procedures. Surface contamination was found in 100% of the tested pharmacy locations in both studies. Cyclophosphamide in the urine has been estimated to increase the risk of cancers in exposed workers. Sessink et al.[5] based their estimate of increased cancer risk (1.4 to 10 additional cases per year per million workers exposed) on daily exposure to cyclophosphamide, with urinary excretion averaging 0.18 μg per 24 hours in pharmacy personnel. This level of exposure is similar to that in 11 other reports of urinary excretion of cyclophosphamide by health care workers (0 to 5.2 μg per 24 hours), summarized by Sessink and Bos.[6] As calculated by Harrison et al.,[7] using the model employed by Sessink et al.,[5] chronic exposure to cyclophosphamide high enough to result in excretion of 17.75 μg per 24 hours, as reported for one worker in the study by Vandenbroucke and Robays,[2] may result in 138–986 additional cancer cases per year per million workers. From the study by Wick et al.,[3] the estimated increased risk of cancer from the reported level of exposure could range from 1.8 to 73 cases per year per million workers.

It is likely that surface contamination presents a risk in most compounding environments.[8] Controlling exposure to hazardous drugs requires a careful process of hazard recognition, risk assessment, development of control measures, communication of the risks and control measures (i.e., quality assurance), and training to ensure that the indicated controls will be utilized.

Environment

Hazardous drugs should be compounded in a controlled area, preferably centralized, where access can be limited to authorized personnel who are trained in handling requirements.[9,10] Drug packages, bins, shelves, and storage areas for hazardous drugs must bear distinctive labels identifying those drugs as requiring special han-

◀ Key Idea ▶

It is likely that surface contamination presents a risk in most compounding environments.

◆ Best Practice ◆
Because of the hazardous nature of these preparations, an environment where air pressure is negative to the surrounding areas is preferred.

dling precautions.[1] Segregation of hazardous-drug inventory from other drug inventory improves control and reduces the number of staff members potentially exposed to the danger.[1] Hazardous drugs should be stored in an area with sufficient general exhaust ventilation to dilute and remove any airborne contaminants.[11] Because of the hazardous nature of these preparations, an environment where air pressure is negative to the surrounding areas is preferred. Positive-pressure environments should be avoided because of the potential spread of contamination from poor technique or spills. Potentially contaminated air from compounding areas should be exhausted to the outside by using appropriate ventilation techniques.

Much of the compounding and administration of hazardous drugs throughout the United States is done in outpatient or clinic settings with the patients and their family members proximal to the mixing area. Therefore, care must be taken to minimize the contamination and to maximize the effectiveness of cleaning (decontamination) activities. Design of such areas must include surfaces that are readily cleaned and decontaminated.

Avoid upholstered and carpeted surfaces, as they are not readily cleaned. Several studies have reported floor contamination and ineffectively cleaned floors and surfaces.[3,4,12,13] Locating break areas and refreshment areas for staff, patients, and others away from areas of potential contamination is critical for reducing unwanted exposure.[1]

Ventilation Controls

Reduction in environmental contamination may be achieved by utilizing one of the recommended ventilation controls.[11] Ventilation or engineering controls are devices designed to eliminate or reduce worker exposures to chemical, biological, radiological, ergonomic, or physical hazards. Ventilation controls also are used to provide the critical environment necessary to compound sterile preparations.

There are several potential sources of contamination. Studies have shown that there may be contamination on the outside of vials received from the manufacturer or distributor[3,14,15] that work practices required to maximize the effectiveness of the Class II biological safety cabinet (BSC) may be unknown or neglected; and that hazardous-drug solutions may vaporize, which makes the effectiveness of the high-efficiency particulate air (HEPA) filter in providing containment questionable.[16–18]

Many studies of surface contamination have discovered deposits of hazardous drugs on the floor in front of the BSC, indicating *possible* escape of drug through the open front of the Class II BSC.[3,4,12,13] In an effort to eliminate and/or reduce the possibility of contamination, employers must install proper ventilation controls. BSCs (Class II and III) and isolators are discussed Chapter 5.

Training

The Federal Hazard Communication Standard (HCS)[19] requires that employers provide safety training to all employees involved in handling hazardous substances. All staff members who handle hazardous drugs must receive safety training that includes recognition of hazardous drugs and appropriate spill response. All individuals transporting hazardous drugs must have safety training that includes spill control and have spill kits immediately accessible. Safety training is required for housekeepers and patient care assistants who handle drug waste and patient waste as well as pharmacists, pharmacy technicians, and nurses who compound and/or administer hazardous drugs.

All staff who will be compounding hazardous drugs must be trained in stringent aseptic and negative-pressure techniques necessary for working with sterile hazardous drugs. Aseptic technique will be covered in Chapter 8. Once trained,

> ◆ **Best Practice** ◆
> **The training should be continually assessed and reinforced.**

staff must demonstrate competence by an objective method, and competency must be reassessed on a regular basis.[9,10]

Emergency Procedures

All areas where hazardous drugs are handled must have spill kits and emergency skin and eye decontamination kits available, as well as relevant material safety data sheets (MSDSs) for guidance. The Federal HCS requires MSDSs to be readily available in the workplace to all employees working with hazardous chemicals (**Appendix 4-1**). More detailed spill control procedures are covered in Chapter 9.

Personal Contamination

Contamination of protective equipment or clothing, or direct skin or eye contact, should be treated by:

- Immediately removing the gloves or gown and disposing in an approved chemotherapy waste container.
- Immediately cleansing the affected skin with soap and water.
- Flooding an affected eye at an eyewash fountain or with water or isotonic eyewash designated for that purpose for at least 15 minutes.
- Obtaining medical attention. Protocols for emergency procedures should be maintained at the designated sites for such medical care. Medical attention should also be sought for inhalation of hazardous drugs in powder form.
- Documenting the exposure in the employee's medical record.

Additional information can be found at http://www.osha.gov/dts/osta/otm/otm_vi/otm_vi_2.html.

Housekeeping and Other Staff

In addition to those personnel who manipulate hazardous drugs, training also must be given to housekeeping, laundry, and janitorial staff. Because accidental exposure is possible, support personnel must receive training on the potential hazards of handling laundry, excreta, and so forth contaminated with hazardous drugs, and on safe work procedures when handling these materials.

Medical Surveillance

All workers who handle hazardous drugs should be routinely monitored in a medical-surveillance program. If such a program is not available at work, workers should inform their private health care providers about possible exposures to hazardous drugs and focus on this exposure during visits for routine medical care. The Occupational Safety and Health Administration (OSHA), the National Institute for Occupational Safety and Health (NIOSH), and the American College of Occupational and Environmental Medicine (ACOEM) recommend medical surveillance as the recognized standard of occupational-health practice for hazardous-drug handlers.[9–11, 20]

Elements of medical-surveillance programs should include the following items:

- Pre-placement histories and medical exams should be conducted to document exposed workers' baseline health status.
- A questionnaire should be developed to collect medical and reproductive history and occupational information. This questionnaire should be used in both the pre-placement examination and ongoing surveillance. Questionnaires should include questions on prior and current employee duties, frequency of drug handling, and information on the amount of drug handled. The answers can be used to estimate the potential intensity of exposure. Special considerations should be given to the reproductive history, including menstrual irregularities, of employees handling hazardous drugs.
- Physical examinations should be completed at the time of hire and then every 1–2 years unless

> ◀ **Key Idea** ▶
>
> **OSHA, NIOSH, and the American College of Occupational and Environmental Medicine recommend medical surveillance as the recognized standard of occupational-health practice for hazardous-drug handlers.**

a worker has a documented incident of overexposure or has a health questionnaire and/or blood work that indicates the need for closer monitoring.

- Specific laboratory studies should include a complete blood count with differential, liver function tests, and urinalysis completed at the time of hire and every 1–2 years.
- After an acute exposure such as a splash or other drug contact with skin or mucous membranes, the physical examination should focus on the exposed areas and the clinical signs of rash or irritation to those areas, as well as the target organs of the hazardous drug involved.
- OSHA recommends worker preparation and administration logs, which provide an objective assessment of possible exposure to hazardous drugs. A review of how often and for how long a worker handles hazardous drugs can be included in the periodic medical exam.
- Follow-up physical examinations and additional laboratory tests are indicated for those workers who have had acute exposures or who have shown health changes during routine monitoring.

SUMMARY

A comprehensive safety program for controlling workplace exposure to hazardous drugs must include environmental and ventilation controls, training, work practices, and personal protective equipment. Such safety programs must be able to identify potentially exposed workers and those who might be at higher risk of adverse health effects from this exposure. All workers who handle hazardous drugs should be routinely monitored in a medical-surveillance program.

REFERENCES

1. ASHP guidelines on handling hazardous drugs. *Am J Health-Syst Pharm*. In press. Refer to http://www.ashp.org/bestpractices/ drugdistribution/Prep_Gdl_HazDrugs.pdf.

2. Vandenbroucke J, Robays H. How to protect environment and employees against cytotoxic agents, the UZ Ghent experience. *J Oncol Pharm Pract.* 2001; 6:146–152.

3. Wick C, Slawson MH, Jorgenson JA, et al. Using a closed-system protective device to reduce personnel exposure to antineoplastic agents. *Am J Health Syst Pharm.* 2003; 60:2314–2320.

4. Sessink PJM, Boer KA, Scheefhals APH, et al. Occupational exposure to antineoplastic agents at several departments in a hospital: environmental contamination and excretion of cyclophosphamide and ifosfamide in urine of exposed workers. *Int Arch Occup Environ Health.* 1992; 64:105–112.

5. Sessink PJM, Kroese ED, van Kranen HJ, et al. Cancer risk assessment for health care workers occupationally exposed to cyclophosphamide. *Int Arch Occup Environ Health.* 1995; 67:317–323.

6. Sessink PJM, Bos RP. Drugs hazardous to healthcare workers: evaluation of methods for monitoring occupational exposure to cyto-static drugs. *Drug Saf.* 1999; 20:347–359.

7. Harrison BR, Peters BG, Bing MR. Comparison of surface contamination with cyclophospha-mide and fluorouracil in three pharmacies using a closed system drug-transfer device versus standard preparation tech-niques. Submitted for publication to *AJHP* August 2005.

8. Kromhout H, Hoek F, Uitterhoeve R, et al. Postulating a dermal pathway for exposure to antineoplastic drugs among hospital workers. Applying a conceptual model to the results of three workplace surveys. *Ann Occup Hyg.* 2000; 44(7):551–560.

9. Controlling occupational exposure to hazard-ous drugs. In: OSHA Technical Manual (OSHA Instruction CPL 2-2.20B CH-4). Washington, DC: Directorate of Technical Support, Occupa-tional Safety and Health Administration; 1995:Chap 21.

10. Controlling occupational exposure to hazard-ous drugs. In: OSHA Technical Manual, TED

1-0.15A. Section VI: Chapter 2. January 20, 1999. Available at: http://www.osha.gov/dts/osta/otm/otm_vi/otm_vi_2.html#2.

11. NIOSH Alert: Preventing Occupational Exposures to Antineoplastic and Other Hazardous Drugs in Healthcare Settings. Atlanta, GA: Centers for Disease Control and Prevention, National Institute for Occupational Safety and Health; 2004. DHHS (NIOSH) publication 2004-165.

12. Connor TH, Anderson RW, Sessink PJM, et al. Surface contamination with antineoplastic agents in six cancer treatment centers in the United Sates and Canada. *Am J Health Syst Pharm.* 1999; 56:1427–1432.

13. Connor TH, Anderson RW, Sessink PJ, et al. Effectiveness of a closed-system device in containing surface contamination with cyclophosphamide and ifosfamide in an IV admixture area. *Am J Health-Syst Pharm.* 2002; 59:68–72.

14. Connor TH, Sessink PJM, Harrison BR, et al. External contamination on chemotherapy drug vials: defining the problem and evaluation of new cleaning techniques. *Am J Health Syst Pharm.* 2005; 62:475–484.

15. Kiffmeyer TK, Ing KG, Schoppe G. External contamination of cytotoxic drug packing: Safe handling and cleaning procedures. *J Oncol Pharm Practice.* 2000; 6:13.

16. Opiolka S, Schmidt KG, Kiffmeyer K, et al. Determination of the vapor pressure of cytotoxic drugs and its effects on occupational safety [Abstract]. *J Oncol Pharm Practice.* 2000; 6:15.

17. Kiffmeyer TK, Kube C, Opiolka S, et al. Vapor pressures, evaporation behavior and airborne concentrations of hazardous drugs: implications for occupational safety. *Pharmaceut J.* 2002; 268:331–337.

18. Connor TH, Shults M, Fraser TP. Determination of the vaporization of solutions of mutagenic antineoplastic agents at 23 and 36° C using a dessicator technique. *Mutat Res.* 2000; 470:85–92.

19. Code of Federal Regulations. Title 29 Hazard Communication Standard CFR 1910-1200. http://www.osha.gov/pls/oshaweb/owadisp.show_document?p_table=STANDARDS&p_id=10099. Accessed November 1, 2004.

20. American College of Occupational and Environmental Medicine (ACOEM).Committee report: ACOEM reproductive hazard management guidelines. *J Occup Environ Med.* 1996; 38(1):83–90.

EXERCISES

1. List the ventilation controls used in your facility to control exposure to hazardous drugs.
2. Identify the safety and work practice training programs available in your facility.
3. Determine who is responsible for the medical surveillance program in your facility.

SELF-ASSESSMENT

1. All workers who handle hazardous drugs should be routinely monitored in a medical-surveillance program.

    A. True.
    B. False.

2. Hazardous drugs should be compounded in an environment where air pressure is positive to the surrounding areas.

    A. True.
    B. False.

3. Which of the following statements about ventilation controls is TRUE?

    A. Ventilation or engineering controls are devices designed to eliminate or reduce worker exposures to chemical, biological, radiological, ergonomic, or physical hazards.

B. Ventilation controls do not provide the critical environment necessary to compound sterile preparations.

4. Only authorized and adequately trained personnel should receive, prepare, transport, or administer hazardous drugs.

A. True.
B. False.

Return to video ▶

Appendix 4-1
Sample Material Safety Data Sheet (MSDS)—GC-764

Section I. CHEMICAL PRODUCT AND COMPANY IDENTIFICATION

PRODUCT: GC-764
SUPPLIER: EMERGENCY 24 HOUR PHONE:

CHEMICAL MANUFACTURER INC.   1 - 800 - 424 - 7659
Rt. 1 Box 21
Hereweare, OK 74056
(918) 749-9118

Section II. COMPOSITION/INFORMATION ON INGREDIENTS

HAZARDOUS COMPONENTS/ CAS NUMBER	EXPOSURE LIMITS		CONCENTRATION (%)
FORMALDEHYDE (50-00-0)	OSHA:	.75 ppm (TWA)	37%
	ACGIH:	.75 ppm (TWA)	
	ACGIH:	2 ppm STEL	Action level 0.5 ppm
METHYL ALCOHOL (67-56-1)	OSHA:	200 ppm PEL(TWA)	7–12%
	ACGIH:	200 ppm (TLV SKIN) (TWA)	
	ACGIH:	250 ppm STEL	

Section III. HAZARDS IDENTIFICATION

ACUTE EXPOSURE: Corrosive to skin, eyes, and mucous membranes.
CHRONIC EXPOSURE: Can cause damage to the eyes, liver, heart, kidneys, and gastrointestinal disturbances. Prolonged contact may cause hardening or tanning of the skin. Formaldehyde is listed as a carcinogen.

Potential Health Effects

EYE: Liquid, vapor or mist causes tearing, severe irritation or burns. High concentration may cause irreversible damage. Methanol ingestion may cause blindness.

SKIN: Causes irritation or drying of the skin.

INHALATION: Causes irritation of the nose and throat with headache. Breathing high concentrations may cause nausea, vomiting, headache, dizziness, and irregular eye movements.

INGESTION: Poisonous if swallowed. May cause nausea, vomiting, dizziness, drowsiness, blurred vision, reduced body temperature, weak irregular pulse, and nervous system effects. May cause burns to mucous membranes. May cause blindness.

CARCINOGENICITY:	NTP:	Yes
	IARC:	Yes
	OSHA:	Yes

Section IV. FIRST AID MEASURES

EYE CONTACT: Flush eyes with water for 15 minutes. Get medical attention if symptoms develop and persist.

SKIN CONTACT: Flush with water or soap and water for 15 minutes or until all traces have been removed. Seek medical attention if symptoms develop and persist.

INHALATION: Remove victim to fresh air and, if needed, immediately begin artificial respiration. Give oxygen if breathing is labored. Get emergency medical help. Contact physician immediately.

INGESTION: Induce vomiting if victim is conscious by giving water, then stick fingers down throat. Give activated charcoal slurry. Get medical attention. Never give unconscious person anything by mouth.

Section V. FIRE FIGHTING MEASURES

FLASHPOINT (METHOD): Approx 140–150 F

FLAMMABLE LIMITS: Lower - 7   Upper - 73

EXTINGUISHING MEDIA: DRY POWDER
CARBON DIOXIDE (CO2)
ALCOHOL FOAM

Special Fire Fighting Procedures: Approach fire from upwind side. Avoid breathing smoke, fumes, mist, or vapors on the downwind side. Firefighters wear protective clothing and self-contained breathing apparatus.

Unusual Fire and Explosion Hazards: Firefighters wear protective clothing, and self contained breathing apparatus. Containers may explode from internal pressure if confined to fire. Cool with water. Keep unnecessary people away.

Section VI. ACCIDENTAL RELEASE MEASURES

Steps To Be Taken In Case Material Is Released Or Spilled:

SMALL SPILLS: Pick up with absorbent media. Store as HAZARDOUS waste.

LARGE SPILLS: Contain with dikes. Pick up with vacuum truck. Handle as HAZARDOUS waste. Notify proper local, state, and federal agencies.

Other Precautions: Clean up leaks immediately to prevent soil or water contamination.

Section VII. HANDLING AND STORAGE

Precautions To Be Taken:

Store away from oxidizers or materials bearing a yellow "D.O.T." label.

Store in a cool, ventilated area.

Store away from ignition sources.

Section VIII. EXPOSURE CONTROLS/PERSONAL PROTECTION

Engineering Controls:

Local exhaust is desired in closed places.
Mechanical exhaust is required to maintain exposure levels below limits.

Personal Protection:

RESPIRATORY PROTECTION: Required for exposure greater than 1 ppm. Cartridge or canister type for formaldehyde if concentration is 1-10 ppm. Industrial canister if concentration is 10–100 ppm.

PROTECTIVE GLOVES: Chemical impervious gloves.

EYE PROTECTION: Chemical goggles or full face shield.

OTHER PROTECTIVE EQUIPMENT: HMIS Personal Protection: X: Boots, aprons, drench showers, eye wash as needed for protection against spills and /or splashes.

WORK HYGIENIC PRACTICES: Avoid contact with skin, eyes, and clothing. After handling this product, wash hands before eating, drinking, or smoking. If contact occurs, remove contaminated clothing. If needed, take First Aid action shown in Section IV. Launder contaminated clothing before reuse.

Section IX. PHYSICAL AND CHEMICAL PROPERTIES

Appearance: Clear Liquid, blend

pH: 2.8–4.0

Melting Point/Melting Range: ND

Vapor Pressure: Approx 40 mm/hg @ 100°F

Solubility: Soluble

Evaporation Rate: ND

Odor: Pungent odor

Boiling Point/Boiling Range: 206–214°F

Flash Point: 140–155°F

Vapor Density: (Air =1) Approx 1.03

Specific Gravity: (H2O=1) 1.075–1.202

Freezing Point: < 32°F

Section X. STABILITY AND REACTIVITY

Chemical Stability: Stable

Materials to Avoid: Extreme temperatures may cause separation and polymerization.

Incompatible Materials: Strong oxidizing substances, strong bases, amines, acids.

Hazardous Decomposition or Byproducts: Formaldehyde, formic acid, oxides of carbon.

Hazardous Polymerization will not occur.

Section XI. TOXICOLOGICAL INFORMATION

Toxicological information is available. Write to address in Section 1.

Section XII. ECOLOGICAL INFORMATION

Ecological data is available for formaldehyde. Write to address in Section 1.

Section XIII. DISPOSAL CONSIDERATIONS

RCRA Hazardous Waste:

D002 - Character of Corrosivity

U154 - Methanol

Waste Disposal Method: EPA approved Hazardous Waste Site. Follow applicable local, state, and federal regulations.

Section XIV. TRANSPORT INFORMATION

DOT (Department of Transportation):

Proper Shipping Name: Formaldehyde Solution

Hazard Class: 3

UN/NA Number: UN1198

Packaging Group: PG III

Reportable Quantity (RQ): RQ required if > 270 pounds.

North American Emergency Response Guidebook (NAERG) #: Guide 132

Section XV. REGULATORY INFORMATION

SARA TITLE III, SECTION 313

In accordance with 40 CFR, 372.45, this product contains the following materials which have been classified as TOXIC under SARA TITLE III, SECTION 313.

TOXIC CHEMICAL	CAS #	CONCENTRATION (%)
Formaldehyde	50-00-0	37%
Methanol	67-56-1	7–12%

SARA TPQ:	None
SARA RQ:	None

EPA HAZARDS:	Acute - Yes
	Chronic - Yes
	Flammability - Yes
	Sudden Release of Pressure - No
	Reactive - No

CERCLA RQ VALUE:	Formaldehyde - 270 pounds
RCRA Hazardous Waste:	D002 - Character of Corrosivity
	U154 - Methanol
Clean Air:	CAA Section 111
Clean Water:	N/A
States Lists:	Massachusetts, New Jersey, Pennsylvania
TSCA, 40 CFR 710:	Sources of the raw materials used in this mixture assure that all chemical ingredients present are in compliance with Section 8(b) Chemical Substance Inventory, or are otherwise in compliance with TSCA.

Section XVI. OTHER INFORMATION

HMIS HEALTH	3
HMIS FLAMMABILITY	2
HMIS REACTIVITY	1
HMIS PERSONAL PROTECTION	X

This MSDS has been revised to upgrade format only. This MSDS will supersede previously issued MSDS.

The data presented is true and correct to the best of our knowledge and belief, however, neither seller nor preparer makes any warranties, express or implied, concerning the information presented. The user is cautioned to perform his own hazard evaluation and to rely upon his own determinations.

Source:

Biological Safety Cabinets

5

Ventilation controls for the safe handling of hazardous drugs include biological safety cabinets (BSCs) and isolators. In Chapter 5, you will review the three classes of BSCs, their specific properties, and their usefulness in the preparation of hazardous drugs.

OBJECTIVES

Upon completion of this chapter, you will be able to:

1. Define the three classes of BSCs.
2. Identify which BSC is best used for handling of hazardous drugs and why.
3. Understand the concerns associated with Class II BSCs.
4. Identify work practices for safe use of Class II BSCs.

DISCUSSION POINTS

The National Institutes of Health divides BSCs into three classes based on their applicability for handling biological (infectious) material.[1,2]

Best Practice

When using a Class II BSC for compounding hazardous drugs, exhaust 100% of the contaminated air through a HEPA filter to the outside whenever feasible and always if the hazardous drug is volatile.

Class I

Class I BSCs are ventilated cabinets for personnel and environmental protection, with unrecirculated inward airflow (i.e., the air flows away from the operator) that exhausts all air to the atmosphere after filtration through a high-efficiency particulate air (HEPA) filter. Class I cabinets are suitable for work where no product protection is required.

Class II

Class II BSCs are ventilated cabinets for personnel, product, and environmental protection. They feature an open front with inward airflow for personnel protection, HEPA-filtered laminar air flow for product protection, and HEPA-filtered exhaust air for environmental protection (**Figure 5-1**).

There are four subclasses of Class II BSCs, according to the type of ventilation requirements: Type A1, Type A2, Type B1, and Type B2.

Type A1

Type A1 cabinets (1) maintain a minimum average inflow velocity of 75 feet per minute (fpm) through the work area access opening; (2) have HEPA-filtered downflow air that is a portion of the mixed downflow and inflow air from a common plenum (i.e., a plenum from which a portion of the air is exhausted from the cabinet and the remainder supplied to the work area); (3) may exhaust HEPA-filtered air back into the work room or to the environment through an exhaust canopy; and (4) may have positive-pressure contaminated ducts and plenums that are not surrounded by negative-pressure plenums.

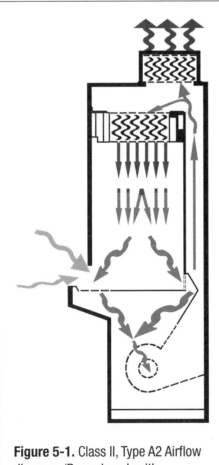

Figure 5-1. Class II, Type A2 Airflow diagram. (Reproduced, with permission, from NuAire, Inc., Plymouth, MN.)

Type A1 cabinets are not suitable for work with volatile toxic chemicals and volatile radionuclides.

Type A2

Type A2 cabinets (1) maintain a minimum average inflow velocity of 100 fpm through the work area access opening; (2) have HEPA-filtered downflow air that is a portion of the mixed downflow and inflow air from a common exhaust plenum; (3) may exhaust HEPA-filtered air back into the work room or to the environment through an exhaust canopy; and (4) have all biologically contaminated ducts and plenums under negative pressure or surrounded by negative-pressure ducts and plenums.

Type A2 cabinets used for work with minute quantities of volatile toxic chemicals and tracer amounts of radionuclides, required as an adjunct to microbiological studies, must be exhausted through properly functioning exhaust canopies.

Type B1

Type B1 cabinets (1) maintain a minimum average inflow velocity of 100 fpm through the work area access opening; (2) have HEPA-filtered downflow air composed largely of uncontaminated recirculated inflow air; (3) exhaust most of the contaminated downflow air through a dedicated duct exhausted to the atmosphere after passing through a HEPA filter; and (4) have all biologically contaminated ducts and plenums under negative pressure or surrounded by negative-pressure ducts and plenums.

Type B1 cabinets may be used for work with minute quantities of volatile toxic chemicals and tracer amounts of radionuclides required as an adjunct to microbiological studies if the work is done in the directly exhausted portion of the cabinet, of if the chemicals and radionuclides will not interfere with the work when recirculated in the downflow air.

Type B2

Type B2 cabinets (1) maintain a minimum average inflow velocity of 100 fpm through the work area access opening; (2) have HEPA-filtered downflow air drawn from the laboratory or the outside air (i.e., downflow air is not recirculated from the cabinet exhaust air); (3) exhaust all inflow and downflow air to the atmosphere after filtration through the HEPA filter without recirculation in the cabinet or return to the laboratory; and (4) have all contaminated ducts and plenums under negative pressure or surrounded by directly exhausted (nonrecirculated through the work area) negative-pressure ducts and plenums.

Type B2 cabinets may be used for work with volatile toxic chemicals and radionuclides required as an adjunct to microbiological studies.

Class III

Class III BSCs are totally enclosed, ventilated cabinets of gas-tight construction. Operations in the cabinet are conducted through attached rubber gloves. The cabinet is maintained under negative air pressure of at least 0.5 inch water gauge. Supply air is drawn into the cabinet through HEPA filters. The exhaust air is treated by double HEPA filtration, or by HEPA filtration and incineration.[1]

BSCs FOR HANDLING HAZARDOUS DRUGS

In the early 1980s, the *Class II BSC* was determined to be more effective than the horizontal laminar-flow workstation in reducing exposure of pharmacy compounding staff to hazardous preparations.[3] Because of its product, environmental, and personnel protection, the Class II BSC has been recommended by the American Society of Health-System Pharmacists (ASHP),[4] the Occupational Safety and Health Administration (OSHA),[5] and the National Institute for Occupational Safety and Health (NIOSH)[6] for compounding sterile preparations of hazardous drugs. The Class II, Type B

◀ **Key Idea** ▶

ASHP, OSHA, and NIOSH include the Class II BSC in their recommendations for compounding sterile preparations of hazardous drugs.

cabinet is preferred due to its outside exhaust. The *Class I BSC* is appropriate only for nonsterile compounding of hazardous drugs, as it offers no product protection. Although OSHA and NIOSH include the *Class III BSC* as an acceptable ventilation control for handling hazardous drugs, the extensive outside exhaust requirements, along with the cost of purchasing and operating the Class III BSC, have resulted in little use of this cabinet.

NIOSH recommends a nonrecirculating BSC (Class II, Type B2 or Class III) for use with drugs that volatilize. Volatile agents pass through HEPA filters and as such will build up in a recirculating device and pass through the exhaust HEPA into the work room. BSC exhausts must be vented to the outside for use with volatile hazardous drugs.

The isolator or ventilated glove box is an alternative to the Class III BSC and will be discussed in Chapter 6.

For the purpose of this lesson, only Class II cabinets will be discussed in detail.

CLASS II BSC

Concerns

Class II BSCs must be equipped with visual and/or auditory gauges that indicate whether appropriate airflows are being maintained. The effectiveness of Class II BSCs in containing contamination may be affected by drafts if equipment is placed near doors, traffic areas, and other air-handling equipment. It is preferable to place the Class II BSC in an area that is limited to handling hazardous drugs.

It is imperative that workers understand and accept that the Class II BSC does not prevent the generation of contamination within the cabinet and that its effectiveness in containing that contamination depends on worker technique. Although studies in the 1980s showed the Class II BSC to be effective, studies in the 1990s, using analytical methods significantly more specific and

---

◄ Key Idea ►

It is imperative that workers understand and accept that the Class II BSC does not prevent the generation of contamination within the cabinet and that its effectiveness in containing that contamination depends on worker technique.

---

sensitive than the Ames test, indicate that environmental and worker contamination occurs in workplace settings despite the use of controls recommended in published guidelines, which include the use of the Class II BSC. The exact cause of contamination has yet to be determined, but the open front of the Class II BSC makes this cabinet very technique dependent.

The Class II BSC, depending on the type, may have recirculating airflow within the cabinet and exhaust of contaminated air back into the work environment through HEPA filters. Once used for hazardous drugs, the Class II BSC is a contaminated environment with contaminated plenums that cannot be reached for surface cleaning. The plenum under the work tray collects room dirt and debris that mixes with hazardous-drug residue when the BSC is operational. Drafts and other laminar airflow equipment placed near the BSC can further damage the containment properties of the inflow air barrier, resulting in contamination of the work environment. To prevent the contamination in the BSC from coming back into the work environment through the open front, the cabinet blower must operate continuously.

If turned off for maintenance, the BSC must first be surface cleaned and decontaminated. The front must be sealed with plastic and taped; a BSC not exhausted to the outside must have the exhaust HEPA housing covered and taped. BSCs should be certified by a qualified technician at least every 6 months. In addition, a technician must recertify the BSC any time the cabinet is repaired or moved.

Work Practices

The use of a Class II BSC must be accompanied by a stringent program of work practices including training, demonstrated competence, contamination reduction, ancillary devices (such as closed-system transfer devices), and decontamination. Without special design considerations,

Class II BSCs are not recommended in traditional, positive-pressure clean rooms where contamination from hazardous drugs may result in airborne contamination that may spread from the open front to surrounding areas.

The Class II BSCs have vertical-flow, HEPA-filtered air as their aseptic environment. Before beginning an operation in a Class II BSC, personnel should wash their hands and put on a pair of chemotherapy gloves and a polyethylene-coated gown, followed by a second pair of chemotherapy gloves. The work surface should be decontaminated with sodium hypochlorite detergent and neutralizer or disinfected with alcohol, depending on when it was last decontaminated.

The front shield of the Class II BSC must be placed appropriately to ensure the effectiveness of the air barrier containment system. Most Class II BSCs are equipped with an alarm system to notify the user if the front shield is not in the correct position. A preparation pad may be used in the Class II BSC during compounding.

The use of a preparation pad in the Class II BSC was found to possibly interfere with the airflow in one study, but was determined to be without consequences to the airflow in another.[7,8] A large pad that might protrude into the front or rear airflows must not be used. As the pad may absorb small spills, it may become a source of contamination for anything placed on it. A preparation pad is not readily decontaminated and must be replaced and discarded after each batch, and frequently during extended batch compounding.

Movement of hands and arms in the Class II BSC has been shown to disrupt the air barrier. Side-to-side movement is especially disruptive. Avoid leaving and reentering the work area of the Class II BSC by assembling all needed drugs and supplies prior to beginning compounding. Only the items needed to compound a dose or batch should be placed in the Class II BSC to reduce contamination on extraneous materials.

Hazardous-drug vials have been shown to be

> ◆ **Best Practice** ◆
> Avoid leaving and reentering the work area of the Class II BSC by assembling all needed drugs and supplies prior to beginning compounding.

contaminated when received. All hazardous-drug vials must be handled with gloves. Wipe down the vials with moist gauze after placing them in the Class II BSC. Contain and discard the gauze as hazardous waste. Change the outer glove prior to continuing.

Intravenous bags and/or bottles may be hung from the bar, if care is taken not to place any sterile objects below them. All items must be placed well within the Class II cabinet, away from the unfiltered air at the front barrier. The containment characteristics of the Class II BSC depend on the airflow through both the front and back grills. Nothing should block the air grills of the BSC. A small waste/sharps container may be placed along the sidewall toward the back of the BSC as long as it does not interfere with the rear grill.

Final preparations also have been shown to be contaminated during the compounding process. Wipe off the final preparations with moist gauze. Change the outer glove prior to flagging the label for final check to avoid transferring contamination to the checker.

The operator of the Class II BSC should be seated such that his/her shoulders are at the level of the bottom of the front shield. This provides face and eye protection while positioning the operator to correctly compound within the cabinet (**Figure 5-2**).

SUMMARY

More information on the design and use of Class II BSCs is available from the National Sanitation Foundation standard 49-04[9] and the ASHP 1990 technical assistance bulletin.[4] Universally, good organization skills and technique are essential to minimize contamination and maximize productivity.

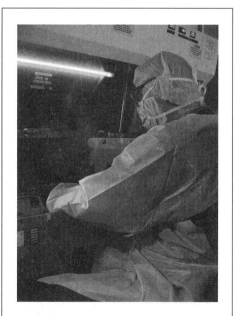

Figure 5-2. The correct position for the operator of a Class II BSC is to be seated with his/her shoulders level to the bottom of the front shield.

REFERENCES

1. National Institutes of Health. NIH Guidelines for Research Involving Recombinant DNA

Molecules. April 2002. Available at: http://
www4.od.nih.gov/oba/rac/guidelines_02/
NIH_Guidelines_Apr_02.htm. Accessed October 13, 2005.

2. Centers for Disease Control and Prevention and National Institutes of Health. Biosafety in Microbiological and Biomedical Laboratories (BMBL). 4th ed. May 1999. Available at: http://www.cdc.gov/od/ohs/biosfty/bmbl4/bmbl4toc.htm. Accessed October 13, 2005.

3. Anderson RW, Pucket WH, Dana WJ, et al. Risk of handling injectable antineoplastic agents. *Am J Hosp Pharm.* 1982; 39:1881–1887.

4. ASHP technical assistance bulletin on handling cytotoxic and hazardous drugs. *Am J Hosp Pharm.* 1990; 47:1033–1049.

5. Controlling occupational exposure to hazardous drugs. In: OSHA Technical Manual, TED 1-0.15A. Section VI: Chapter 2. January 20, 1999. Available at: http://www.osha.gov/dts/osta/otm/otm_vi/otm_vi_2.html#2.

6. NIOSH Alert: Preventing Occupational Exposures to Antineoplastic and Other Hazardous Drugs in Healthcare Settings. Atlanta, GA: Centers for Disease Control and Prevention, National Institute for Occupational Safety and Health; 2004. DHHS (NIOSH) publication 2004-165.

7. Minoia C, Turci R, Sottani C, et al. Application of high performance liquid chromatography/tandem mass spectrometry in the environmental and biological monitoring of health care personnel occupationally exposed to cyclophosphamide and ifosfamide. *Rapid Commun Mass Spectrom.* 1998; 12:1485–1493.

8. Peters W. Containment capabilities of a Class II, Type A2 BSC using a chemo pad on the worksurface. [Personal communication] Minneapolis, MN: Technical Bulletin from NuAire, Inc.; June 2, 2003.

9. NSF/ANSI Standard 49-04: Class II (laminar flow) biosafety cabinetry. NSF International Standard/American National Standard Institute standard. NSF International. Ann Arbor, MI: National Sanitation Foundation; 2002. Revised 2004.

EXERCISES

1. Assemble all necessary supplies for use in a Class II BSC for compounding one dose of a hazardous drug.
2. Practice decontaminating final preparations by using moist gauze and changing the outer glove.

SELF-ASSESSMENT

1. Why is the Class II BSC preferred for compounding sterile preparations of hazardous drugs?

   A. Provides personnel protection.
   B. Provides product protection.
   C. Provides environmental protection.
   D. All of the above.

2. All hazardous drug vials must be handled with gloves.

   A. True.
   B. False.

3. Class II BSCs are recommended in traditional, positive-pressure clean rooms.

   A. True.
   B. False.

4. The effectiveness of Class II BSCs in containing contamination may be affected by drafts due to placement of equipment near doors, traffic areas, and other air-handling equipment.

   A. True.
   B. False.

5. Which of the following statements is incorrect?

    A. Containment of contamination within the cabinet of Class II BSCs is technique dependent.

    B. Class II BSCs should be placed in an area limited to handling hazardous drugs.

    C. The Class II BSC provides complete protection in containing hazardous drugs.

Return to video ▶

6

Isolators

Ventilation controls for the safe handling of hazardous drugs include biological safety cabinets (BSCs) and compounding aseptic isolators (CAIs) or isolators. In Chapter 6, you will review isolator or glove box technology and specific practices in using an isolator for handling hazardous drugs.

OBJECTIVES

Upon completion of this chapter, you will be able to:

1. Define the basic components of an isolator.
2. List the concerns associated with isolators for handling hazardous drugs.
3. Identify work practices for safe use of isolators when compounding hazardous drugs.

DISCUSSION POINTS

History

Isolation technology was first developed by the nuclear industry to handle radioactive materials without exposing personnel to radiation. The technology was adopted by the electronics industry to protect their products from exposure to the workers. The pharmaceutical application of isolators has been well documented in industry and was initially used in hospital pharmacy in the United Kingdom more than 20 years ago. The isolator's ability to protect both the preparation and the worker are important for the handling of hazardous drugs. The National Institute for Occupational Safety and Health (NIOSH) Alert on hazardous drugs specifies that only ventilated cabinets may be used to handle either sterile or nonsterile hazardous drugs.[1] Therefore, only those isolators, or glove boxes, that are ventilated provide appropriate control. Currently, there is no uniformly accepted definition of an isolator, thus clouding the selection process.

Definition of Isolator

One definition of an isolator is a controlled environment with fixed walls, floor, and ceiling.[2] Transfers of materials in and out of the environment are done using gloves, sleeves, and airlocks that prevent the internal environment from being exposed to the surrounding environment's conditions of air quality. An isolator that may be used for handling hazardous drugs also requires an air-handling system, which provides the required ventilation. The NIOSH Alert further defines isolators as "containment" or "aseptic containment" depending on the need to compound sterile or nonsterile preparations.[1] The aseptic-containment isolator provides both an aseptic environment to allow sterile compounding and a contained environment to protect personnel and the work area from contamination. All ventilated cabinets, including isolators, must be equipped with a continuous-monitoring device that confirms adequate airflow.

High-efficiency particulate air (HEPA) filters must be used to exhaust air from the isolator. Isolators that exhaust 100% of the filtered air to the outside are preferred. Ventilated isolators that recirculate air inside the cabinet or exhaust air back into the room environment should not be used unless the hazardous drugs are nonvolatile.

The internal environment of the isolator can be pressurized to be either positive or negative to the surrounding environment. Positive pressure in the isolator is recommended for compounding sterile preparations, protecting the internal environment from microbial contamination. However, this positive pressure may allow hazardous-drug contamination to escape into the surrounding environment if there is a breach in the isolator's main chamber. One solution to the requirement for both positive and negative pressurization is the use of an exhausted transfer or interchange chamber that is negative to the isolator main chamber and negative to the surrounding environment.

Concerns

As with the Class II BSC, the isolator does not prevent generation of contamination during the compounding process. The effectiveness of the isolator in containing that contamination depends on how the isolator is designed, the technique of the operator, and a thorough understanding of the potential ways that contamination generated in the main isolator chamber may be brought out into the environment.

Use of an isolator must be accompanied by a stringent program of work practices including training, demonstrated competence, contamination reduction, ancillary devices (such as closed-system transfer devices), and decontamination. Contamination from the main chamber of the isolator may be brought into the workroom environment through the transfer, interchange chamber and on the surfaces of items placed in and removed from the isolator (final preparation). Appropriate sanitizing of drugs and supplies placed into the transfer, interchange chamber—coupled with wipe down of final preparation before removal from antechamber—is essential to reduce contamination of the work room from the isolator.

Recirculating isolators depend on HEPA filters, which may not be sufficient to remove volatile hazardous-drug contamination from the airflow. Isolators discharging contaminated air into the work room through HEPA filters are no more effective than nonvented Class II BSCs if the contamination vaporizes. The NIOSH Alert recommends nonrecirculating, externally vented units for hazardous drugs that are volatile.[1]

Work Practices

The aseptic environment in the isolator is achieved by HEPA-filtered air as either laminar flow (unidirectional) or turbulent flow and sanitization of the isolator surfaces with an appropriate antimicrobial agent. All surfaces of the isolator should be easily reachable by a worker using the fixed-glove assembly. Surface cleaning must be done using the gloves. Isolators used for handling hazardous drugs must be routinely decontaminated (i.e., surface contamination from hazardous drugs must be removed or deactivated) while the isolator is in a sealed state. Many isolators are equipped with fronts that may be opened for cleaning. Opening an isolator used for hazardous drugs allows any surface contamination to be moved into the environment. Avoid opening the front of a contaminated isolator and thoroughly decontaminate the isolator with detergent and a deactivating agent before performing any operation that requires opening the front.

Because contamination of the work area is possible when hazardous drugs or surrogates are being handled in isolators,[3] use of gowns while

◀ Key Idea ▶

To reduce workroom contamination, it is essential that drugs are compounded appropriately, and the preparation is wiped down before removal from the interchange chamber.

◆ Best Practice ◆ Isolators used for handling hazardous drugs must be routinely decontaminated while the isolator is in a sealed state.

performing operations with or within isolators is prudent. To reduce transfer of bodily contamination from one worker to another, a pair of disposable gloves, appropriate for handling hazardous drugs, should be worn within the fixed-glove assembly.

Workers cleaning and or decontaminating an isolator should wear a pair of appropriate, disposable gloves and a polyethylene-coated gown before accessing the main chamber through the fixed-glove assembly. Cleaning and/or decontaminating the transfer, interchange chamber or antechamber of a negative-pressure isolator may be done through the chamber door, wearing two pairs of gloves and a gown. The antechamber of a positive-pressure isolator should be decontaminated from the main chamber using the fixed-glove assembly. The operator must wear disposable gloves and a gown.

Isolators equipped with vertical laminar flow, HEPA-filtered supply air require the same compounding techniques with respect to the critical sites as a Class II BSC. Intravenous bags and/or bottles may be hung from the bar if care is taken not to place any sterile objects below them. The operator's hands must not obstruct the filtered air flow during compounding.

Initial Inspection

Ideally, the isolator should be certified to an industry standard. However, no such standard currently exists. The Controlled Environment Testing Association has recently developed a guidance document for the use of isolators in health care facilities.[4]

Prior to any operation in an isolator, perform the following checks:

1. Inspect the fixed-glove assembly for tears or damage. If the gloves are not intact, replace the damaged glove using the manufacturer's specified technique. The sleeve assembly is less prone to damage, but the operator must ensure

that the sleeve is undamaged and that the connection to the isolator and the connection to the glove are intact.

2. Inspect all gauges that indicate readiness of the isolator and exhaust system. Do not use the isolator if all gauges do not indicate that the isolator is ready to use. If the isolator has been turned off, allow the blower to run for the time specified by the manufacturer prior to utilizing the isolator for compounding hazardous drugs.

Before beginning an operation in an isolator, take the following safety precautions:

1. Personnel should wash their hands and put on a pair of appropriate gloves and a polyethylene-coated gown.
2. The interior of the isolator and the transfer, interchange chamber or antechamber should be decontaminated with detergent, sodium hypochlorite, and neutralizer. Then, they should be thoroughly rinsed with sterile water and/or disinfected with alcohol, depending on when they were last decontaminated. Decontamination is required following any spill in the isolator during compounding. Chlorinated materials may damage stainless steel if allowed to remain on the surface without neutralization and rinsing.

Working in the Isolator

It is common practice to sanitize drugs and supplies either before placing them in the isolator transfer chamber or antechamber or while they are in the transfer chamber, to reduce the transfer of particulate and microbial contamination into the isolator main chamber. Equally important in compounding hazardous drugs is to prevent the transfer of hazardous-drug contamination. Hazardous-drug vials have been shown to be contaminated when received. All hazardous-drug vials must be handled with two pairs of gloves. Wipe down the vials with moist gauze when placing

◆ **Best Practice** ◆
Perform all safety precautions before beginning an operation in an isolator.

them into the transfer or interchange chamber. Contain and discard the gauze as hazardous waste. Change the outer glove prior to continuing.

A preparation pad may be used in the isolator provided it does not interfere with any air grills. The pad must be placed in the transfer chamber, then brought into the main chamber using the fixed-glove assembly. As the pad may absorb small spills, it may become a source of contamination for anything placed on it. A preparation pad cannot readily be either decontaminated or sanitized. The addition of a pad into a sterile compounding area may compromise the cleanliness of the preparation chamber. If used with hazardous drugs, the preparation pad must be replaced and discarded after each batch, and frequently during extended batch compounding. The preparation pad must be contained in a sealable plastic bag and discarded as hazardous waste.

Assemble all supplies, solutions, and equipment necessary to complete the preparation or batch. Place only those items needed to compound a dose or batch in the transfer or interchange chamber. Limit the number of doses per batch to what can be comfortably placed in the isolator and still be clearly delineated as one dose. Avoid placing unnecessary items in the main chamber of the isolator to reduce contamination on extraneous materials. Do not place tranport bags in the main chamber of the isolator.

Decontaminate the gloves of the fixed-glove assembly before the first batch or preparation of the day and after each batch with sodium hypochlorite and neutralizer. Wipe off the gloves with gauze moistened with sterile water. Gloves should be sanitized frequently during batch operations with an appropriate disinfectant.

Using the fixed-glove assembly, open the door to the transfer chamber or antechamber and sanitize or decontaminate the materials by spraying or wiping them off with an appropriate agent. Transfer the drugs, solutions, and supplies from the transfer chamber to the main chamber.

Preparation of hazardous drugs in an isolator requires stringent aseptic technique with or without the use of closed-system transfer devices. Sharps contaminated with hazardous drugs must be discarded into a small waste container placed inside the main chamber of the isolator, or discarded into the attached waste containers if the isolator is so equipped. Hazardous drug-contaminated material may be placed into sealable, thick plastic bags for discard into hazardous-drug waste containers.

Syringes and solutions must remain in the isolator for checking. The operator must aid the checker in determining the contents of all syringes prior to completing the compounding. The checker must don gloves if accessing the isolator main chamber through the fixed-glove assembly.

Final preparations also have been shown to be contaminated during the compounding process. Wipe off the fixed-glove assembly and the final preparations with moist gauze prior to flagging the label for final check. The checked preparation must be placed and sealed into a transport bag by a worker wearing clean gloves.

Seal and then decontaminate surfaces of waste/sharps containers before removing them from the isolator through the transfer chamber. Following completion of a dose or a batch, let the isolator run for several minutes without operator activity to allow the air to be exhausted and the isolator purged of contaminated air. Once the air is purged, remove all materials through the transfer chamber and decontaminate the interior surfaces of the main chamber and the transfer chamber. Check grills and diffusers for any spilled or splashed material and decontaminate appropriately.

SUMMARY

Isolators are currently in limited use for handling hazardous drugs. The lack of industry standard for an isolator and the variety of available designs make selection and use of an isolator problematic.

Advantages of an isolator include the closed cabinetry, the restricted access to the main chamber, and the improved ability to decontaminate the compounding area. Disadvantages include the fact that the isolator, similar to the Class II BSC, does not prevent the generation of contamination and must be used with a vigorous program of meticulous technique and work practices, along with frequent decontamination to prevent transfer of hazardous drugs from the main compounding chamber to the surrounding environment.

REFERENCES

1. NIOSH Alert: Preventing Occupational Exposures to Antineoplastic and Other Hazardous Drugs in Healthcare Settings. Atlanta, GA: Centers for Disease Control and Prevention, National Institute for Occupational Safety and Health; 2004. DHHS (NIOSH) publication 2004-165.
2. Rahe H. Isolators. In: Buchanan EC, Schneider P, eds. Compounding Sterile Preparations. 2nd ed. ASHP, Bethesda, MD: American Society of Health-System Pharmacists; 2005:chap 4.
3. Mason HJ, Blair S, Sams C, et al. Exposure to antineoplastic drugs in two UK hospital pharmacy units. *Ann Occup Hyg*. October 2005; 49:603–10.
4. CETA Applications Guide for the Use of Compounding Isolators in Compounding Sterile Preparations in Healthcare Facilities. CAG-001-2005. November 8, 2005. http://www.cetainternational.org/reference/Applications GuideBarrierIsolator110805.pdf

EXERCISES

1. Assess the readiness of an isolator for compounding. Check the glove assembly, the sleeve, and the gauges.
2. Practice decontaminating the interior of the isolator and the transfer, antechamber, or interchange chamber.

3. Practice decontaminating gloves using sterile water.

SELF-ASSESSMENT

1. There is no need to use gowns or ancillary devices when compounding hazardous drugs in an isolator.

   A. True.
   B. False.

2. It is common practice to sanitize drugs and supplies either before placing them into the isolator transfer chamber or while they are in the transfer chamber, to reduce the transfer of particulate and microbial contamination into the isolator main chamber.

   A. True.
   B. False.

3. Which of the following statements is incorrect?

   A. Surface cleaning in the isolator must be done using gloves.
   B. Hazardous-drug vials are never contaminated upon receipt.
   C. Isolators are currently in limited use for handling hazardous drugs.

4. Which of the following statements is most accurate?

   A. Workers should wear gloves and a gown to clean the transfer or interchange chamber of a negative-pressure isolator.
   B. Workers should wear a disposable gown to clean the transfer chamber.
   C. Workers should wear two pairs of disposable gloves and a gown when cleaning the transfer chamber.

5. Currently, there is no uniformly accepted definition of an isolator.

    A. True.

    B. False.

Return to video ▶

Personal Protective Equipment

7

In Chapter 7, you will review a number of recommendations for wearing personal protective equipment (PPE). The equipment should include well-fitted disposable American Society for Testing and Materials (ASTM) tested-gloves, an appropriate protective gown, and eye protection and/or a face shield for some indications.

OBJECTIVES

Upon completion of this chapter, you will be able to:

1. Identify the appropriate PPE needed for safe handling of hazardous drugs during compounding, administration, disposal, and spill containment.
2. Review current recommendations regarding use of PPE for safe handling of hazardous drugs during compounding.
3. Describe recommended procedures regarding use of PPE for safe handling of hazardous drugs during administration.
4. Describe recommended procedures regarding use of PPE for safe handling of hazardous drugs during disposal.

DISCUSSION POINTS

Engineering and administrative controls, and proper PPE, may protect workers from exposures to hazardous drugs. Personal protective equipment must be provided to all employees handling hazardous drugs.

Gloves

Gloves are essential for handling hazardous drugs. Only gloves that have been tested against the ASTM standard for resistance to chemotherapy should be used for handling hazardous drugs.[1] Gloves must be worn at all times when handling drug vials, performing inventory control procedures, and assembling hazardous drugs and supplies for compounding either a batch or a single dose.

During compounding in a Class II biological safety cabinet (BSC), gloves and gowns are required to prevent skin surfaces from contacting hazardous drugs. New studies on gloves indicate that many latex and nonlatex materials provide effective protection against penetration and permeation by most hazardous drugs.[2-6] Recent concerns about latex sensitivity have prompted testing of newer glove materials. Gloves made of nitrile, neoprene, and polyurethane have been successfully tested against a battery of antineoplastic drugs by several researchers.[4-6] The ASTM has developed testing standards for assessing the resistance of medical gloves to permeation by chemotherapy drugs.[1] Gloves that meet this testing standard earn the designation of "chemotherapy gloves." Gloves selected for use with hazardous drugs should meet this ASTM standard. Connor and Xiang studied the effect of isopropyl alcohol on the permeation of latex and nitrile gloves exposed to antineoplastic agents.[7] During the limited study period of 30 minutes, they found that the use of isopropyl alcohol for cleaning and decontaminating did not appear to affect the integrity of either material.

◀ **Key Idea** ▶

Gloves must be worn at all times when handling drug vials, performing inventory control procedures, and assembling hazardous drugs and supplies for compounding either a batch or a single dose.

In most glove test systems, the glove material is static, as opposed to the stressing and flexing that glove material receives during actual use. In a study designed to examine permeation under static and flexed conditions, no significant difference in permeation was reported, except in thin latex examination gloves.[8] However, a second study that used a cotton glove under the latex glove detected permeation of antineoplastics through latex gloves during actual working conditions.[9]

The breakthrough time for cyclophosphamide was only 10 minutes. The authors speculate that the cotton glove may have acted as a wick, drawing the hazardous drug contamination through the outer glove. Nonetheless, under actual working conditions, double gloving and wearing gloves no longer than 30 minutes are prudent practices. Permeability of gloves to the hazardous drugs has been shown to depend on the drug, the gloving material, the thickness of the gloves, and the exposure time. Powder-free gloves are preferred both to avoid contamination of the sterile processing area with powder particulates and to prevent absorption of contaminants by the powder, resulting in the potential for increased dermal contact. Hands should be thoroughly washed before putting on gloves and after removing them. Care must be taken in removing gloves.

Several studies indicate that contamination of the outside of gloves is common following compounding and that this contamination on the outside may be spread to other surfaces during the compounding process.[10–14] Studies also indicate that this contamination may lead to dermal absorption by workers not actively involved in the compounding and administration of hazardous drugs.[9,10]

The use of two pairs of gloves is recommended for compounding. The outer glove should be removed once compounding has been completed and the final preparation wiped off. The inner glove is worn to affix labels and place the prepara-

> ◆ **Best Practice** ◆
> **Powder-free gloves are preferred both to avoid contamination of the sterile environment and to prevent absorption of contaminants by powder, resulting in the potential for increased dermal contact.**

tion into a sealable containment bag for transport. (Note: Transport bags must never be placed in the BSC during compounding to avoid inadvertent contamination of the outside surface of the bag.) During batch compounding, gloves should be changed at least every 30 minutes. Gloves (at least the outer glove) must be changed whenever it is necessary to come out of and reenter the BSC. For protection of the preparation, the outer glove should be sanitized when reentering the BSC. Gloves also must be changed immediately if torn, punctured, or contaminated.

When two pairs of gloves are used, one pair is worn under the gown cuff and the second pair is placed over the cuff. When the gloves are removed, the contaminated glove fingers must touch only the outer contaminated surface of the glove, never the inner surface. If the inner glove becomes contaminated, then both pairs of gloves must be changed. When removing any PPE, care must be taken to avoid putting contamination into the environment. Both the inner and outer gloves should be considered contaminated, and glove surfaces must never touch the skin or any surface that may be touched by the unprotected skin of others. Gloves should be placed in a sealable plastic bag for containment prior to disposal.

Class III BSCs and isolators are equipped with attached gloves or gauntlets. They should be considered contaminated once the cabinet or isolator has been used for compounding hazardous drugs. Contamination from the gloves/gauntlets may be transferred to the surfaces of all items within the cabinet. Gloves/gauntlets must be surface-cleaned after compounding is complete. Staff, wearing clean gloves to avoid spreading the contamination, must wipe off all final preparations. In one report on isolator use for handling hazardous drugs, the author noted that an additional pair of powder-free, nonlatex gloves was worn during compounding.[15]

> ◆ **Best Practice** ◆
> **Gloves/gauntlets must be surface cleaned after compounding is complete.**

Glove Recommendations

■ Select powder-free, good-quality gloves made of latex, nitrile, polyurethane, neoprene, or other materials that are labeled as Chemo Gloves.

■ Inspect gloves for visible defects.

■ Wear double gloves for any handling of hazardous drugs.

■ The National Institute for Occupational Safety Alert recommends double gloves for all activities involving hazardous drugs.[16]

■ The Oncology Nursing Society also recommends double gloving for administration.[17]

■ Change gloves every 30 minutes during compounding, or immediately when damaged or contaminated.

■ Change gloves after administering a dose of hazardous drug or when leaving the immediate administration area.

■ Remove outer glove after wiping down the final preparation but before labeling or removing the preparation from the BSC.

■ In an isolator, gloves/gauntlets must be surface-cleaned after compounding is complete and the final preparation has been wiped down.

■ Don fresh gloves to remove the final preparation from pass-through, label, and place in clean transport bag.

■ Wash hands before putting on gloves and after removing gloves.

■ Remove gloves with care to avoid contamination.

■ Contain and dispose of contaminated gloves as hazardous waste.

Gowns

Gowns or coveralls are used in the compounding of sterile preparations to avoid inadvertent contamination with particulates from the clothes or skin of workers. Guidelines for the safe handling of hazardous drugs recommend the use of gowns for compounding in the BSC, or isolator; during administration, spill control, and waste management to protect the worker from hazardous-drug contamination by any residue generated during the handling process.[16–19]

Early recommendations for barrier protective gowns required that they be disposable and made of a lint-free, low-permeability fabric with a closed front, long sleeves, and tight-fitting elastic or knit cuffs.[18] Washable garments, such as lab coats, scrubs, and cloth gowns, absorb fluids and provide no barrier to hazardous-drug absorption.

Recent studies into the ability of disposable gowns to resist penetration by hazardous drugs found variation in the protection provided by the commercially available materials. In an evaluation of polypropylene-based gowns, Connor found that polypropylene spunbond nonwoven material alone and polypropylene-polyethylene copolymer spunbond provided little protection against penetration by a battery of aqueous and nonaqueous hazardous drugs.[20] Various constructions of polyethylene (e.g., spunbond/meltblown/spunbond) result in materials that are completely impermeable or only slightly permeable to hazardous drugs. Connor noted that these coated materials are similar in appearance to several other nonwoven materials but perform differently and that workers could expect to be protected from exposure for up to 4 hours when using the coated gowning materials. Harrison and Kloos reported similar findings in a study of 6 disposable gowning materials and 15 hazardous drugs.[21] Only gowns with polyethylene or vinyl coatings provided adequate splash protection and prevented penetration of the hazardous drugs.

In a subjective assessment of worker comfort, the more protective gowns were found to be warmer and thus less comfortable. These findings agree with an earlier study that found that the most protective gowning materials were the most uncomfortable to wear.[22] The lack of comfort could cause resistance to behavioral change.

Researchers have looked at gown contamination with fluorescent scans, and high-performance liquid chromatography and tandem mass spectrometry.[14,23] In one study, researchers scanned nurses and pharmacists wearing gowns during compounding and administration of hazardous drugs.[23] Of a total of 18 contamination spots detected, 5 were present on the gowns of nurses after drug administration. No spots were discovered on the gowns of pharmacists after compounding.

In contrast, researchers[14] using a more sensitive assay placed pads in various body locations, both over and under the gowns used by the subjects during compounding and administration of cyclophosphamide and ifosfamide. Workers wore short-sleeved nursing uniforms, disposable or cotton gowns, and vinyl or latex gloves. More contamination was found during compounding than during administration. Contamination found on the pads placed on the arms of preparers is consistent with the design and typical work practices used in a Class II BSC where the hands and arms are extended into the contaminated work area of the cabinet. Remarkably, one preparer had contamination on the back of the gown, indicating possible touch contamination with the Class II BSC during removal of final preparation.

Although early guidelines did not contain a maximum length of time that a gown should be worn, Connor's work supports a 2- to 3-hour window for a coated gown.[20] Contamination of gowns during glove changes must be a consideration. If the inner pair of gloves requires changing, a gown change should be considered. Gowns worn during compounding as barrier protection against hazardous drugs must never be worn outside the immediate compounding area. Gowns worn during administration should be changed when leaving the patient care area and immediately if contaminated. Gowns are to be disposed of after removal to avoid being a source of contamination to other staff and the environment.

Gown Recommendations

1. Select disposable gowns of material tested to be protective against hazardous drugs.

> ◆ **Best Practice** ◆
> **Consider changing your gown if you must change your inner pair of gloves.**

2. Coated gowns must be worn no longer than 3 hours during compounding and changed immediately when damaged or contaminated.
3. Gowns must be worn during administration of hazardous drugs.
4. Remove gowns with care to avoid contamination.
5. Dispose of gowns immediately upon removal.
6. Contain and dispose of contaminated gowns as hazardous waste.
7. Wash hands after removing and disposing of gown.

Additional Personal Protective Equipment

Eye and Facial Protection

Eye and face protection should be used whenever there is a possibility of exposure from splashing or uncontrolled aerosolization of hazardous drugs (e.g., while containing a spill or handling a damaged shipping carton). In these instances, a face shield, rather than safety glasses or goggles, is recommended due to the improved skin protection afforded by the shield.

Similar circumstances warrant the use of a respirator. All workers who may utilize a respirator must be fit-tested and trained to use the appropriate respirator according to the Occupational Safety and Health Administration Respirator Standard.[24,25] The appropriate respirator must be available at all times.

Surgical masks may be required in a controlled environment to provide additional protection against contamination of the preparation. These masks, however, do not provide worker protection. An appropriate respirator will do both.

Shoe and Hair Coverings

Shoe and hair coverings should be worn during the compounding process to minimize particulate contamination of the controlled work zone and the preparation.[26] With the potential for hazardous-drug contamination on the floor in the compounding and administration areas, shoe coverings also

> ◆ **Best Practice** ◆
> A face shield, rather than safety glasses or goggles, is recommended whenever there is a risk of splashing or uncontrolled aerosolization of drugs due to the improved skin protection afforded by the shield.

are recommended as contamination-control mechanisms. As such, shoe coverings must be removed, while wearing gloves, when leaving the compounding area. Gloves should be worn and care must be taken when removing hair or shoe coverings to prevent contamination from spreading to clean areas. Hair and shoe coverings used in the hazardous-drug areas must be sealed in plastic bags, along with used gloves, and discarded as hazardous waste.

Touch Contamination

There are many possible causes of touch contamination. Direct observation of pharmacists and technicians during drug preparation and handling may yield information about potential sources of contamination. Unless actual sources of surface contamination are identified, they cannot be eliminated.

The following work practices are likely to result in decreased touch contamination.

■ Compound all hazardous drugs in one pharmacy or centralized drug preparation area.
■ Gather all necessary supplies before beginning work in the Class II BSC.
■ Change gloves every 30 minutes and whenever contamination occurs.
■ Wash hands after removing gloves for any reason and prior to donning new gloves.
■ Place waste generated in the Class II BSC (e.g., outer gloves, vials, gauze) in a sealed plastic bag before removing it from the Class II BSC.
■ Discard the sealed bag containing contaminated material and equipment in a puncture-proof hazardous-drug waste receptacle placed immediately outside the Class II BSC.
■ For isolators, use a waste containment and disposal system specific to the type of isolator in use.
■ Never access a sealed hazardous-drug transport bag without wearing gloves.
■ Visually examine the contents of the sealed bag. If visible leakage is present, do not open the

bag. To reduce the risk of touch contamination, dose verification can occur at the administration site.

- Use luer-locking connections on all intravenous (IV) delivery devices.
- Use needleless systems whenever possible.
- Use and dispose of sharps carefully.
- Avoid spiking IV bags or bottles that contain hazardous drugs. Attach and prime all tubing in the pharmacy with nondrug solution before adding hazardous drugs or back-prime with plain solution.
- Never "unspike" IV bags or bottles. Disconnect and discard infusion bags and bottles with tubing intact.
- Place hazardous-drug disposal containers near the workspace.
- Keep the lid closed on hazardous-drug disposal containers except when placing contaminated materials into the containers.
- Hazardous-drug contaminated materials should never be forced into waste containers. Be sure there is sufficient space in the container to drop the contaminated material into it.
- Clean BSC, isolator, and countertops or table tops in the mixing area with a two-step cleaning method such as SurfaceSafe™ daily, after all other contaminated materials are removed from the area.

SUMMARY

Health care workers who work with hazardous drugs are at risk for exposure to the negative side effects associated with these agents. The health risk depends on the toxicity of the drug and the amount of exposure experienced. The probability of health care workers experiencing adverse effects from hazardous drugs increases with the frequency and degree of exposure and the level of deployment of safe workplace practices. Use of PPE is an important component of an overall workplace safety program that should include environmental controls for areas handling hazardous drugs, use of closed systems to prevent release of hazardous drugs into the environment, use of BSCs or barrier isolators to contain any hazardous material that is released, and appropriate deployment of PPE.

REFERENCES

1. American Society for Testing and Materials (ASTM) D 6978-05 Standard Practice for Assessment of Resistance of Medical Gloves to Permeation by Chemotherapy Drugs. West Conshohocken, PA: ASTM; 2005.
2. Connor TH. Permeability testing of glove materials for use with cancer chemotherapy drugs. *Oncology*. 1995; 52:256–259.
3. Singleton LC, Connor TH. An evaluation of the permeability of chemotherapy gloves to three cancer chemotherapy drugs. *Oncol Nurs Forum*. 1999; 26:1491–1496.
4. Gross E, Groce DF. An evaluation of nitrile gloves as an alternative to natural rubber latex for handling chemotherapeutic agents. *J Oncol Pharm Practice*. 1998; 4:165–168.
5. Connor TH. Permeability of nitrile rubber, latex, polyurethane, and neoprene gloves to 18 antineoplastic drugs. *Am J Health-Syst Pharm*. 1999; 56:2450–2453.
6. Klein M, Lambov N, Samev N, et al. Permeation of cytotoxic formulations through swatches from selected medical gloves. *Am J Health-Syst Pharm*. 2003; 60:1006–1011.
7. Conner TH, Xiang Q. The effect of isopropyl alcohol on the permeation of gloves exposed to antineoplastic agents. *J Oncol Pharm Practice*. 2000; 6:109–114.
8. Colligan SA, Horstman SW. Permeation of cancer chemotherapeutic drugs through glove materials under static and flexed conditions. *Appl Occup Environ Hyg*. 1990; 5:848–852.
9. Sessink PJM, Cerna M, Rossner P, et al. Urinary cyclophosphamide excretion and chromosomal aberrations in peripheral blood lymphocytes after occupational exposure to antineoplastic agents. *Mutation Res*. 1994; 309:193–199.

10. Sessink PJM, Boer KA, Scheefhals APH, et al. Occupational exposure to antineoplastic agents at several departments in a hospital: environmental contamination and excretion of cyclophosphamide and ifosfamide in urine of exposed workers. *Int Arch Occup Environ Health.* 1992; 64:105–112.

11. Sessink PJM, Van de Kerkhof MCA, Anzion RB, et al. Environmental contamination and assessment of exposure to antineoplastic agents by determination of cyclophosphamide in urine of exposed pharmacy technicians: is skin absorption an important exposure route? *Arch Environ Health.* 1994; 49:165–169.

12. Sessink PJM, Wittenhorst BCJ, Anzion RBM, et al. Exposure of pharmacy technicians to antineoplastic agents: reevaluation after additional protective measures. *Arch Environ Health.* 1997; 52:240–244.

13. Ensslin AS, Stoll Y, Pethran A, et al. Biological monitoring of cyclophosphamide and ifosfamide in urine of hospital personnel occupationally exposed to cytostatic drugs. *Occup Environ Med.* 1994; 51:229–233.

14. Minoia C, Turci R, Sottani C, et al. Application of high performance liquid chromatography/tandem mass spectrometry in the environmental and biological monitoring of health care personnel occupationally exposed to cyclophosphamide and ifosfamide. *Rapid Commun Mass Spectrom.* 1998; 12:1485–1493.

15. Tillet L. Barrier isolators as an alternative to a cleanroom. *Am J Health-Syst Pharm.* 1999; 56:1433–1436.

16. NIOSH Alert: Preventing Occupational Exposures to Antineoplastic and Other Hazardous Drugs in Healthcare Settings. Atlanta, GA: Centers for Disease Control and Prevention, National Institute for Occupational Safety and Health; 2004. DHHS (NIOSH) publication 2004-165.

17. Polovich M, White J, Kelleher L. Chemotherapy and Biotherapy Guidelines and Recommendations for Practice. 2nd ed. Pittsburgh, PA: Oncology Nursing Society; 2005.

18. ASHP technical assistance bulletin on handling cytotoxic and hazardous drugs. *Am J Hosp Pharm.* 1990; 47:1033–1049.

19. American Society of Health-System Pharmacists. ASHP guidelines on handling hazardous drugs. *Am J Health-Syst Pharm.* In press. Refer to http://www.ashp.org/bestpractices/drugdistribution/Prep_Gdl_HazDrugs.pdf.

20. Connor TH. An evaluation of the permeability of disposable polypropylene-based protective gowns to a battery of cancer chemotherapy drugs. *Appl Occup Environ Hyg.* 1993; 8:785–789.

21. Harrison BR, Kloos MD. Penetration and splash protection of six disposable gown materials against fifteen antineoplastic drugs. *J Oncol Pharm Practice.* 1999; 5:61–66.

22. Laidlaw JL, Connor TH, Theiss JC, et al. Permeability of four disposal protective-clothing materials to seven antineoplastic drugs. *Am J Hosp Pharm.* 1985; 42:2449–2454.

23. Labuhn K, Valanis B, Schoeny R, et al. Nurses' and pharmacists' exposure to antineoplastic drugs: findings from industrial hygiene scans and urine mutagenicity tests. *Cancer Nurs.* 1998; 21:79–89.

24. U.S. Department of Labor. Occupational Safety and Health Administration. Respiratory Protection Standard. 29 CFR 1910.134. Electronic Code of Federal Regulations (e-CFR) http://ecfr.gpoaccess.gov/. Accessed November 1, 2004.

25. Summary for respirator users. National Institute for Occupational Safety and Health (NIOSH). Available at http:// www.cdc.gov/niosh/respsumm.html. Accessed September 15, 2005.

26. Pharmaceutical Compounding - Sterile Preparations. Chapter 797: United States Pharmacopeia (USP). 28th ed. U.S. Pharmacopeial Convention, Inc. Rockville, MD: U.S. Pharmacopeial Convention, Inc.; 2004:2461–2477.

EXERCISES

1. List the seven gowning recommendations outlined in this chapter.
2. Perform the tasks necessary for proper gowning and gloving in preparation for the manipulation of hazardous drugs.

SELF-ASSESSMENT

1. What two statements about gloving for handling hazardous drugs are most accurate?

   A. Wear a single pair of gloves while compounding.
   B. Change gloves every 4 hours.
   C. Change gloves after administering a dose of hazardous drugs.
   D. Sanitize gloves to remove final preparation from pass-through.

2. Gloves must be worn at all times while performing inventory control procedures for hazardous drugs.

   A. True.
   B. False.

3. When dealing with hazardous drugs, surgical masks provide adequate worker protection.

   A. True.
   B. False.

4. To avoid exposure to splashing or uncontrolled aerosolization of hazardous drugs, which type of face protection is recommended?

   A. A face shield.
   B. Safety glasses or goggles.
   C. Mask.
   D. Respirator.

5. Hair and shoe coverings used in the hazardous-drug areas must be sealed in plastic bags and discarded as hazardous waste.

    A. True.
    B. False.

Return to video ▶

8

Aseptic Technique

In Chapter 8, you will identify a number of techniques that compounding personnel should use to limit exposure to hazardous drugs. In addition, this chapter includes a discussion on the need for ongoing training and competency testing to ensure that personnel are skilled and knowledgeable enough to prevent exposure and maintain containment when handling hazardous drugs.

OBJECTIVES

Upon completion of this chapter, you will be able to:

1. Define proper aseptic technique in the handling of hazardous drugs.
2. Explain the need for specialized training for personnel working with hazardous drugs.
3. Recognize acceptable work practices for handling hazardous drugs.

DISCUSSION POINTS

Aseptic technique describes the methods used to manipulate sterile preparations so that they remain sterile.[1,2] Technique is a separate element in the compounding of sterile preparations, independent from equipment and the environment. When performed accurately, negative-pressure aseptic technique minimizes the escape of drug from vials and ampuls.[3] Needleless devices have been developed to reduce health care workers' risk of exposure to blood-borne pathogens. None of these devices have been tested for reduction of hazardous-drug contamination. The appropriateness of these devices in the safe handling of hazardous drugs is unproven.

Vials

When hazardous drugs are reconstituted in vials, it is critical to avoid pressurizing the contents of the vial, which can cause drug to spray out from around the needle, aerosolizing the drug into the work area of the biological safety cabinet (BSC) or negative-pressure isolator. To minimize or prevent pressurization, the compounding personnel can utilize techniques to create a slight negative pressure in the vial. Too much negative pressure, however, can cause leakage from the needle when it is withdrawn from the vial.

When hazardous-drug solutions are manipulated with a syringe, several recommended safe-handling techniques should be utilized. They are:

- No more than three quarters (75%) of the syringe's volume should be filled with the solution. This safe-handling technique minimizes the risk of the plunger separating from the syringe barrel.
- Once the diluent is drawn up, the needle should be inserted into the vial and the plunger pulled back and air is drawn into the syringe. Small amounts of diluent should be transferred slowly as equal volumes of air are removed.

◀ **Key Idea** ▶

To minimize or prevent overpressurization, use techniques to create a slight negative pressure in the vial.

The needle should be kept in the vial, and the contents should be swirled carefully until dissolved. With the vial inverted, the proper amount of drug solution should be gradually withdrawn while equal volumes of air are exchanged for solution.

■ The exact volume of drug needed must be measured while the needle is in the vial, and any excess drug should remain in the vial. With the vial in the upright position, a small amount of air should be drawn through the needle and just to the hub of the syringe. The hub should be clear before the needle is removed.

■ If a hazardous drug is transferred to an intravenous (IV) bag, care must be taken to puncture only the septum of the injection port and avoid puncturing the sides of the port or the bag.

■ After the drug solution is injected into the IV bag, the IV port, container, and set should be wiped with moist gauze. The final preparation should be labeled, including an auxiliary warning, and the injection port covered with a protective shield or a tamper-evident seal. Clean gloves should be used to place the final container into a sealable bag to contain any leakage.

Ampuls

Ampuls are composed entirely of glass. Once an ampul is broken, it becomes an open-system, single-use container. Because air or fluid may now pass freely in and out of the ampuls, the volume of fluid removed does not have to be replaced with air.

Before an ampul is opened, any solution visible in the top portion (head) should be moved to the bottom (body) by one of the following methods:

■ Swirling the ampul in an upright position.
■ Tapping the head with one's finger.
■ Inverting the ampul and then quickly swinging it into an upright position.

To open an ampul properly, its neck should be cleansed with an alcohol swab and the swab should be left in place. This swab can prevent accidental cuts to the fingers as well as spraying of glass particles and aerosolized drug. The head of the ampul should be held between the thumb and index finger of one hand, and the body should be held with the thumb and index finger of the other hand. Pressure should be exerted on both thumbs, pushing away from oneself in a quick motion to "snap" the ampul open at the neck. Ampuls should not be opened toward the high-efficiency particulate air (HEPA) filter of the laminar airflow workbench or toward other sterile preparations within the workbench. Extreme pressure may result in crushing the head between the thumb and index finger. Therefore, if the ampul does not open easily, it should be rotated so that pressure on the neck is at a different angle.

To withdraw medication from an ampul, it should be tilted and the bevel of the needle placed in the corner space (or shoulder) near the opening. Surface tension should keep the solution from spilling out of the tilted ampul. The syringe plunger is then pulled back to withdraw the solution.

The use of a filter needle (e.g., a needle with a 5-μm filter in the hub) eliminates fragments of glass or paint that may have fallen into the solution from being drawn up into the syringe. Sometimes, a medication (e.g., a suspension) may need to be withdrawn from an ampul with a regular needle; a filter needle should then be used to push the drug out of the syringe. In all cases, the same filter needle should not be used for both withdrawing and injecting, because that will nullify the filtering effort.

Training and Demonstration of Competence

All staff members who will be compounding hazardous drugs must be trained in aseptic techniques necessary for working with sterile hazardous drugs. Once trained, staff must demonstrate competence by an objective method, and competency must be reassessed on a regular basis.[4]

> ◆ **Best Practice** ◆
> Open an ampul by first cleansing the neck with an alcohol swab. Leave the swab in place to prevent accidental cuts to the fingers.

A written program must be in place to address how training will be developed, delivered, and evaluated. Elements of this program include:

- Information on any operation/procedure used in a work area containing hazardous drugs.
- Training methods involving a surrogate drug that may be visually monitored.
- The measures employees can take to protect themselves from hazardous drugs (including appropriate work practices, emergency procedures, and personal protective equipment [PPE]), and hazard communication training.

Knowledge and competence of personnel should be evaluated after the first orientation or training session and at least annually thereafter. Evaluation may involve direct observation of an individual's performance on the job. Nonhazardous solutions may be used for evaluation of preparation techniques. Fluorescein, which will fluoresce under ultraviolet light, provides an easy mechanism for evaluation of technique—and a way to mix technique with training.[5]

Safe-Handling Work Practices

Written safe-handling work practices or specific instructions need to be part of the written quality-assurance plan. These procedures should be formulated or otherwise adapted from existing written/published procedures. Employers must train workers on the procedures and make this training available to all personnel involved in the compounding and/or administration of the hazardous drugs. Workers should learn their work site's specific procedures for safe handling.

Although health care workers are most likely to be exposed to hazardous drugs during drug compounding and administration, recent studies suggest that drug residues can be found on the external surfaces of vials.[6–8] Safe-handling practices must be used from the time the drug enters the facility until its disposal (which includes the proper disposal of patients' solid and liquid waste).

Hazardous drugs should be compounded in a properly functioning Class II or III BSC or negative-pressure isolator by staff who have been trained in safety and handling precautions. All PPE should offer proven barrier protection from the hazardous drugs being used. Manufacturers of PPE should be able to provide documentation of the testing performed against various chemical agents. Contaminated PPE and other non-reusable equipment must be disposed of in properly labeled, leak-proof containers. All employees handling hazardous drugs must be able to clean up a spill. The spills in clinical areas cannot wait for a Haz-Mat team.

Manufacturers are beginning to make safety systems to capture escaping liquid or airborne droplets released when IV ports and vials are accessed to prepare the drug.[9-11] These devices are not available for ampuls or glass IV bottles and are not for all drugs or vial sizes.

Vaporized hazardous drugs pose more complex problems than aerosols. Because gases or vapors are not trapped by HEPA filters, ventilation systems must be tailored to exhaust gases or vapor waste safely and properly.

SUMMARY

Proper negative-pressure aseptic technique is an acquired skill. *Pharmacists, technicians, and all those who compound and/or administer hazardous drugs must be trained in and demonstrate competence in negative-pressure aseptic technique before they are allowed to handle these drugs.* Just as safe devices can prevent needlestick exposures, correct practice of aseptic technique may be one of the most effective ways to curb hazardous-drug exposures. In addition to proper gowning, hand washing, and proper use of the BSC or isolator, strict aseptic technique is critical in preventing contamination due to exposure to hazardous drugs.

REFERENCES

1. Buchanan EC, Schneider P, eds. Compounding Sterile Preparations. 2nd ed. Bethesda, MD: American Society of Health-System Pharmacists; 2005.

2. Wallace L. Basics of Aseptic Technique Video Training Program. Bethesda, MD: American Society of Health-System Pharmacists. Publication date: March 2006.

3. Wilson JP, Solimando DA. Aseptic technique as a safety precaution in the preparation of antineoplastic agents. *Hosp Pharm.* 1981; 15:575–581.

4. Controlling occupational exposure to hazardous drugs. In: OSHA Technical Manual, TED 1-0.15A. Section VI: Chapter 2. January 20, 1999. Available at: http://www.osha.gov/dts/osta/otm/otm_vi/otm_vi_2.html#2.

5. Harrison BR, Godefried RJ, Kavanaugh EA. Quality-assurance testing of staff pharmacists handling cytotoxic agents. *Am J Health-Syst Pharm.* 1996; 53:402–407.

6. Sessink PJM, Boer KA, Scheefhals APH, et al. Occupational exposure to antineoplastic agents at several departments in a hospital. *Int Arch Occup Environ Health.* 1992; 64:105–112.

7. Kiffmeyer TK, Ing KG, Schoppe G. External contamination of cytotoxic drug packing: safe handling and cleaning procedures. *J Onc Pharm Practice.* 2000; 6:13.

8. Connor, TH, Sessink, PJM, Harrison BR, et al. External contamination on chemotherapy drug vials: defining the problem and evaluation of new cleaning techniques. *Am J Health-Syst Pharm.* 2005; 62:475–484.

9. Connor TH, Anderson RW, Sessink PJ, et al. Effectiveness of a closed-system device in containing surface contamination with cyclophosphamide and ifosfamide in an I.V. admixture area. *Am J Health-Syst Pharm.* 2002; 59:68–72.

10. Vandenbroucke J, Robays H. How to protect environment and employees against cytotoxic agents, the UZ Gent experience. *J Onc Pharm Practice.* 2001; 6:146–152.

11. Spivey S, Connor TH. Determining sources of workplace contamination with antineoplastic drugs and comparing conventional IV drug preparation with a closed system. *Hosp Pharm*. 2003; 38:135–9.

EXERCISES

1. Using the steps outlined in this chapter, practice opening an ampul in the Class II BSC or isolator.
2. Using diluents only, practice adding and withdrawing fluids from a vial as if you were reconstituting hazardous drugs in vials. Be sure fluids do not leak outside the vial.

SELF-ASSESSMENT

1. Ampuls should be opened toward the HEPA filter of the laminar airflow workbench.

   A. True.
   B. False.

2. Which of the following statements about reconstituting hazardous drugs is (are) correct? Select all that apply.

   A. Pressurize the contents of the vial before withdrawing with a syringe.
   B. Create a slight negative pressure in the vial to avoid aerosolizing the drug.
   C. Too much negative pressure can cause leakage from the needle when it is withdrawn from the vial.
   D. Use a syringe that is no more than half (50%) full when filled with the solution.
   E. Remove the needle from the vial before swirling any contents.

3. When withdrawing a medication from an ampul, you should tilt the ampul and place the bevel of the needle in the shoulder space near the opening.

    A. True.
    B. False.

4. How often should knowledge and competence evaluations be performed? Select the best answer.

    A. At first orientation.
    B. At first orientation and at least once a month.
    C. At first orientation and at least once a year.
    D. Once a month.
    E. Once a year.

5. If a spill occurs in a clinical area, employees should immediately call Haz-Mat and wait for the team to arrive.

    A. True.
    B. False.

Return to video ▶

9

Decontamination, Waste Disposal, and Spill Control

In Chapter 9, you will explore the various tasks and responsibilities involved in handling decontamination, disposing of waste, and cleaning up hazardous spills.

OBJECTIVES

Upon completion of this chapter, you will be able to:

1. Define decontamination.
2. Describe best practices for the containment of hazardous drugs.
3. Explain methods used for disposal of hazardous drugs and contaminated materials.
4. List procedures used to clean up hazardous spills.

◀ **Key Idea** ▶

Surface contamination of the work environment may lead to exposure of workers in the environment.

DISCUSSION POINTS

Contamination of the work environment may occur during any contact with hazardous drugs, including receipt of broken vials, drug contamination on the vial surface, compounding and administration of the drug, handling patient waste, handling drug waste, and disposing of contaminated materials. Surface contamination of the work environment may lead to exposure of workers in the environment.

Strict compliance with policies and procedures related to the storage, handling, compounding, and disposal of hazardous drugs will reduce the number of incidents of environmental contamination, as well as the risk of occupational exposure to these agents.

Decontamination

Decontamination may be defined as cleaning or deactivating. Using alcohol to disinfect the biological safety cabinet (BSC) or isolator will not deactivate any hazardous drugs and may result in the spreading of contamination rather than any actual cleaning.[1,2] Many drug manufacturers recommend the use of sodium hypochlorite bleach as an appropriate deactivating agent for some hazardous drugs.[3] Researchers have shown that strong oxidizing agents (e.g., sodium hypochlorite bleach) are effective deactivators of many of the hazardous drugs.

SurfaceSafe® is a commercially available product that provides a solution of sodium hypochlorite bleach with detergent on one towelette of a two-pack system. The second pack contains thiosulfate to neutralize the bleach and deactivate several of the drugs that do not oxidize readily (e.g., platinum-containing drugs). SurfaceSafe® is designed for use in a Class II BSC but also may be used in a Class III cabinet or an isolator. The bleach is a disinfectant and reduces the need for alcohol.

Containment of Hazardous Drugs

In 1976, the U.S. Environmental Protection Agency (EPA) enacted the Resource Conservation and Recovery Act (RCRA) to provide a mechanism for tracking hazardous waste from its generation to disposal.[4] These regulations apply to drugs (pharmaceuticals), as well as chemicals discarded by pharmacies, hospitals, clinics, and other commercial entities. The RCRA includes lists of agents that are to be considered hazardous waste.

The P list and U list include several drugs that, regardless of concentration, are designated as hazardous wastes if they are the sole active ingredients. This discussion will be limited only to those drugs that are compounded as sterile preparations. P-listed wastes are termed acutely hazardous and include epinephrine, nitroglycerine, and physostigmine. U-listed wastes are toxic, flammable, corrosive, or reactive. Pharmaceuticals on the U list are generally toxic and include cyclophosphamide. In addition to the P and U lists, EPA also designates four characteristics of a hazardous waste: ignitability, toxicity, corrosivity, and reactivity.[5,6]

Once hazardous waste has been identified, it must be collected and stored according to specific EPA and Department of Transportation requirements. Properly labeled, leak-proof, and spill-proof containers made of nonreactive plastic are required for areas where hazardous waste is generated. Hazardous-drug waste may be initially contained in thick, sealable plastic bags before being placed in approved hazardous-waste containers. Needles and any glass fragments should be contained in small, puncture-resistant sharps containers, to be placed into larger containers approved for temporary storage.

Waste contaminated with blood or other body fluids must not be mixed with hazardous waste.

Transport of waste containers from satellite accumulation sites to storage sites must be done by individuals who have completed the hazardous-waste awareness training mandated by the Occu-

---

◆ **Best Practice** ◆
Many drug manufacturers recommend the use of sodium hypochlorite bleach as an appropriate deactivating agent for many hazardous drugs.

pational Safety and Health Administration (OSHA). Hazardous waste must be properly manifested and transported by a federally permitted hazardous-waste transporter to a federally permitted hazardous-waste storage, treatment, or disposal facility. A licensed contractor may be hired to manage the hazardous-waste program.

The waste generator, however, may be held liable for mismanagement of hazardous waste. Investigation of a contractor, including verification of possession and type of license, should be completed and documented before a contractor is engaged. More information on hazardous-waste disposal is available at http://www.hercenter.org.

Disposal of Hazardous Drugs and Contaminated Materials

Hazardous waste must be handled separately from other medical waste to ensure that those individuals handling the waste are protected from potential exposure. Most hazardous waste vendors are not permitted to manage regulated medical waste (RMW or infectious waste). Organizations should check carefully with their hazardous waste vendors to ensure acceptance of all possible hazardous waste, including mixed infectious waste, if needed.

Hazardous wastes are substances that are listed as toxic by the EPA or possess one or more of the following characteristics: acute toxicity, ignitability, corrosivity, or reactivity. Certain hazardous drugs become hazardous wastes when they require disposal. Many other hazardous drugs have characteristics similar to those listed drugs. Although their disposal is not subject to the same regulations, safe-handling precautions still apply.

Hazardous-drug waste containers must be available in all areas where hazardous drugs are prepared and administered. The waste containers should be puncture proof, have a lid that seals securely, and be labeled with an appropriate

◀ **Key Idea** ▶

Safe-handling precautions apply to the disposal of hazardous wastes.

warning. The warning label identifies the contents as hazardous so that the individuals transporting the waste are alerted to the need for special handling. The container should be distinctly different from other types of waste containers (e.g., those used for infectious waste) and should be used only for hazardous-drug waste. Plastic bags (e.g., the sealable bag used for drug transport) may be used to collect hazardous waste, but these should then be placed inside a rigid waste container so that all waste is essentially "double bagged." Keep the lid closed on hazardous-drug disposal containers except when placing contaminated materials into the containers. These practices reduce the risk of drug vapors being released into the environment.

Any item that comes in contact with a hazardous drug during its compounding or administration is considered potentially contaminated and must be disposed of as hazardous waste. Such items include needles, syringes, empty drug vials, ampuls, intravenous (IV) tubing, IV bags or bottles, connecting devices, gauze, and alcohol wipes. Such items should be discarded intact to reduce the possibility of dispersing drug droplets. *Crushing or clipping needles is prohibited.*

Sharp or breakable items must be placed in a puncture-proof container. Use of protected needle devices for intramuscular or subcutaneous injections of hazardous drugs is highly recommended. A disposal container should be present at the site of drug administration to eliminate the need to transport an exposed needle. This recommendation also applies when discontinuing an IV access device with an exposed needle.

Personal protective equipment (PPE) such as gowns, gloves, or face shields worn during drug handling should be disposed of in a hazardous-waste container. Reusable items that have been contaminated should be handled while wearing PPE and cleansed with soap, water, and bleach where appropriate before returning to use.

Avoid overfilling disposal containers. Health care workers should not reach into hazardous-

> ◆ **Best Practice** ◆
> **Hazardous-drug waste containers should be distinctly different from other types of waste containers (e.g., those used for infectious waste) and should be used only for hazardous-drug waste.**

waste containers when discarding contact material. Seal waste containers when three fourths full. Once they are sealed, notify the appropriate personnel to remove the waste containers from the compounding or administration area. Only individuals trained in Haz-Mat response who wear appropriate PPE and who have completed OSHA-mandated hazardous-waste awareness training[8] are allowed to handle the hazardous-drug waste containers.

Hazardous drug-related wastes should be handled separately from other hospital trash. Waste must be stored in a secure area in covered, leak-proof containers or drums with distinct labels such as "CAUTION: HAZARDOUS WASTE." Only licensed disposal contractors may transport hazardous waste from the facility for final disposal. Such contractors must meet local, state, and federal requirements as determined by the EPA. The actual disposal must be performed according to federal, state, and local ordinances. This disposal is done in an EPA-licensed RCRA incinerator. All those involved in hazardous-drug disposal must maintain records related to the transport and disposal.

Spill Management

Policies and procedures must be developed to attempt to prevent spills and to manage spill cleanup of hazardous drugs. Written procedures must specify who is responsible for spill management and must address the size and scope of the spill. Spills must be contained and cleaned up *immediately* by trained workers.

Spill kits containing all of the materials needed to clean up spills of hazardous drugs should be assembled or purchased. These kits should be readily available in all areas where hazardous drugs are routinely handled. The drug handler must obtain a spill kit if hazardous drugs are prepared or administered in a nonroutine area (e.g., a home setting, an unusual patient-care area).

The kit should include sufficient supplies to absorb a spill of about 1000 mL (the volume of one IV bag or bottle). The kit also should contain appropriate PPE to protect the worker during clean up.

A kit should include:

- Two pairs of disposable gloves (one outer pair of heavy, utility gloves and one inner pair of latex or other gloves).
- Nonpermeable, disposable protective garments (coveralls or gown and shoe covers).
- Face shield.
- Absorbent, plastic-backed sheets or spill pads.
- Disposable toweling.
- At least two sealable thick, plastic, hazardous-waste disposal bags (prelabeled with an appropriate warning label).
- A disposable scoop for collecting glass fragments.
- A puncture-resistant container for glass fragments.
- Signs to warn of restricted access to the spill area.

All workers who may be required to clean up a hazardous-drug spill must be trained for this responsibility, including training in how to use PPE and respirators certified by the National Institute for Occupational Safety and Health (NIOSH). OSHA requires a complete respiratory protection program, including fit-testing, for all workers who may be required to use a respirator. Appropriate respirators must be available.

The circumstances and handling of spills should be documented. Health care personnel exposed to hazardous drugs during spill management also should complete an incident report or exposure form. All spill materials must be disposed of as hazardous waste.

Spill Cleanup Procedure

- Only trained workers with appropriate PPE and respirators should attempt to manage a hazardous-drug spill.

- Assess the size and scope of the spill. Call for trained help if necessary.
- Post signs to limit access to spill area.
- Obtain spill kit and respirator.
- Don PPE, including inner and outer gloves and respirator.
- Once fully garbed, contain spill using spill kit supplies.
- Carefully remove any fragments of broken glass and place them in a puncture-resistant container.
- Absorb liquids with spill pads.
- Absorb powder with damp disposable pads or soft toweling.
- Spill cleanup should proceed progressively from areas of lesser to greater contamination.
- Completely remove and place all contaminated material in the disposal bags.
- Rinse the area with water and then clean with detergent and/or hypochlorite bleach and neutralizer.
- Rinse the area several times, and place all materials used for containment and cleanup in disposal bags. Seal these bags and then place them in the appropriate final container for disposal as hazardous waste.
- Carefully remove all PPE using the inner gloves. Place all disposable PPE into disposal bags, seal the bags, and then place them into the appropriate final container.
- Remove inner gloves, contain them in a small, sealable bag, and place the bag into the appropriate final container for disposal as hazardous waste.
- Wash hands thoroughly with soap and water.

Spills in a BSC or Isolator

- Spills occurring in the BSC or isolator should be cleaned up immediately.
- Obtain a spill kit if the volume of the spill exceeds 150 mL or the contents of one drug vial or ampul.
- Wear utility gloves to remove broken glass in a Class II BSC.

- In an isolator, use utility gloves over the fixed glove assembly. In a negative-pressure isolator, fasten the utility gloves to the fixed glove with tape. Care must be taken not to damage the fixed glove assembly when handling broken glass.
- Place glass fragments in the puncture-resistant container located in the BSC or discard into the appropriate waste receptacle of the isolator.
- Thoroughly clean and decontaminate the BSC or isolator.
- Clean and decontaminate the drain spillage trough located under the Class II BSC or isolator, if so equipped.
- If the spill results in liquid being introduced onto the high-efficiency particulate air (HEPA) filter, or powdered aerosel contaminating the "clean side" of the HEPA filter, use of the BSC of isolator should be suspended until the equipment has been decontamintated and the HEPA filter replaced.

SUMMARY

Contamination of the work environment may occur anytime during the normal workday. If contamination is not dealt with swiftly and correctly, workers may be exposed to hazardous drugs. Facilities must follow strict policies and procedures related to the storage, handling, preparation, and disposal of these drugs. Good safety practices will reduce the number of incidents of contamination and protect workers from potential exposure to any hazardous materials.

REFERENCES

1. Sessink PJM, Boer KA, Scheefhals APH, et al. Occupational exposure to antineoplastic agents at several departments in a hospital: environmental contamination and excretion of cyclophosphamide and ifosfamide in urine of exposed workers. *Int Arch Occup Environ Health*. 1992; 64:105–112.
2. Dorr RT, Alberts DS. Topical absorption and

inactivation of cytotoxic anticancer agents in vitro. *Cancer.* 1992; 70(suppl):983–987.

3. Johnson EG, Janosik JE. Manufacturers' recommendations for handling spilled antineoplastic agents. *Am J Hosp Pharm.* 1989; 46:318–319.

4. The Resource Conservation and Recovery Act of 1976. Public Law No. 42, US Code, Chapter 6901-692k.

5. Characteristics of Hazardous Waste. Code of Federal Regulations Title 40, Part 261.20-24. *Federal Register.* May 19, 1980.

6. Characteristics of Hazardous Waste. Code of Federal Regulations Title 40, Part 261.24 (Characteristic of Toxicity). *Federal Register.* March 29, 1990.

7. Healthcare Environmental Resource Center www.hercenter.org - section on Regulated Medical Waste.

8. Hazard material training: Initial Training. Code of Federal Regulations, Part 1910.120(e)(3)(i), Title 29. Electronic Code of Federal Regulations (e-CFR) http://ecfr.gpoaccess.gov/. Accessed November 1, 2004. Emergency Response to Hazardous Substances Releases. CFR Part 1910.120(q)(1-6), Title 29. Electronic Code of Federal Regulations (e-CFR); http://ecfr.gpoaccess.gov/. Accessed November 1, 2004.

EXERCISE

Check your facility's hazardous-drug spill kit. Does the kit have all the recommended elements? When was the last time the kit was inspected?

SELF-ASSESSMENT

1. Written procedures must specify who is responsible for spill management and must address the size and scope of the spill.

   A. True.
   B. False.

2. Which BEST describes the proper use of a waste container for the disposal of hazardous waste?

   A. Hazardous-waste containers are needed only in areas where hazardous drugs are prepared.
   B. Hazardous-waste containers should be the same as other types of waste containers in the area.
   C. Seal hazardous-waste containers when completely full.
   D. Hazardous-waste containers should be puncture proof, have a sealable lid, and have a warning label.

3. When removing PPE, it is recommended to use the outer gloves once they are washed and disinfected.

   A. True.
   B. False.

4. Spill kits are required in compounding facilities but not home care settings.

   A. True.
   B. False.

5. Only licensed disposal contractors may transport hazardous waste from the facility for final disposal.

   A. True.
   B. False.

Return to video ▶

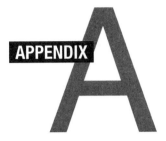

Additional Guidelines

Additional guidelines that address hazardous drugs or the equipment in which they are manipulated include the following:

- *Centers for Disease Control (CDC) and National Institutes of Health (NIH).* Primary Containment for Biohazards [CDC/NIH 2000]. Provides guidance on the selection, installation, testing, and use of BSCs.
- *NIH.* Recommendations for the Safe Handling of Cytotoxic Drugs [NIH 2002]. Includes recommendations for the safe preparation and administration of cytotoxic drugs.
- Polovich M, White JM, Kelleher LO, eds. Chemotherapy and Biotherapy Guidelines and Recommendations for Practice. 2nd ed. Pittsburgh, PA: Oncology Nursing Society; 2005.
- *Oncology Nursing Society.* Safe Handling of Hazardous Drugs [Polovich 2003]. Includes proper handling guidelines for hazardous drugs.
- *United States Pharmacopoeia.* Chapter <797> Pharmaceutical Compounding—Sterile Preparations [USP 2004]. Details the procedures and requirements for compounding sterile preparations and sets standards applicable to all settings in which sterile preparations are compounded.
- *NSF/ANSI Standard 49-04: Class II (laminar flow) biosafety cabinetry.* NSF International standard/American National Standard Institute standard. NSF International. Ann Arbor, MI: National Sanitation Foundation, 2002; revised 2004.
- *PDA.* Technical Report No. 34: Design and Validation of Isolator Systems for the Manufacturing and Testing of Health Care Products [PDA 2001]; a supplemental publication to the PDA Journal of Pharmaceutical Science and Technology. Provides definitions, design, and operation and testing guidance for types of isolators used in the health care product manufacturing industry.
- *American Glovebox Society (AGS).* Guidelines for Gloveboxes; 2nd edition [AGS 1998]. Provides guidance on the design, testing, use, and decommissioning of glovebox containment systems.

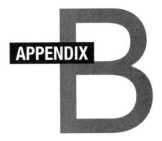

Glossary

A

Aseptic Preparation or Aseptic Processing
The technique involving procedures designed to preclude contamination (of drugs, packaging, equipment, or supplies) by microorganisms during processing.

B

Batch Preparation
Compounding of multiple sterile preparation units, in a single discrete process, by the same individuals, carried out during one limited time period.

Biohazard
An infectious agent presenting a real or potential risk to humans and the environment.

C

Carcinogen
Any cancer-producing substance.

Chemotherapy
The treatment of disease by chemical means; first applied to use of chemicals that affect the causative organism unfavorably but do not harm the patient; currently used to describe drug (chemical) therapy of neoplastic diseases (cancer).

Chemotherapy Drug
A chemical agent used to treat diseases. The term usually refers to a drug used to treat cancer.

Chemotherapy Glove
A medical glove that has been tested by the American Society for Testing and Materials (ASTM) D 6978-05 Standard Practice for Assessment of Resistance of Medical Gloves to Permeation by Chemotherapy Drugs. West Conshohocken, PA: ASTM; 2005.

Chemotherapy Waste

Discarded items such as gowns, gloves, masks, IV tubing, empty bags, empty drug vials, needles and syringes, and other items generated while compounding and administering antineoplastic agents.

Chemotherapy waste may be defined as bulk or trace using the guidelines developed by NIH. (For more information, see ASHP guidelines on handling hazardous drugs. *Am J Health-Syst Pharm*. In press. Refer to http://www.ashp.org/bestpractices/drugdistribution/Gdl_HazDrugs.pdf.)

From guidelines:

Trace-contaminated hazardous drug waste. By the NIH definition of trace chemotherapy waste, "RCRA-empty" containers, needles, syringes, trace-contaminated gowns, gloves, pads, empty IV sets, etc. may be collected and incinerated at a regulated medical waste incinerator. Sharps used in the preparation of hazardous drugs should not be placed in red sharps containers or needle-boxes, since these are most frequently disinfected by autoclaving or microwaving, not by incineration, and pose a risk of aerosolization to waste-handling employees.

Bulk hazardous drug waste. While not official, the term "bulk hazardous drug waste" has been used to differentiate containers that have held either 1) RCRA-listed or characteristic hazardous waste or 2) any hazardous drugs, which are not RCRA empty, or any materials from hazardous drug spill cleanups. These wastes should be managed as hazardous waste.

Clean Room

A room (1) in which the concentration of airborne particles is controlled; (2) that is constructed and used in a manner to minimize the introduction, generation, and retention of particles inside the room; and (3) in which other relevant variables (i.e., temperature, humidity, and pressure) are controlled as necessary.

Clean Zone

Dedicated space (1) in which the concentration of airborne particles is controlled; (2) that is constructed and used in a manner that minimizes the introduction, generation, and retention of particles inside the zone; and (3) in which other relevant variables (i.e., temperature, humidity, and pressure) are controlled as necessary. This zone may be open or enclosed and may or may not be located within a clean room.

Closed System

A device that does not exchange unfiltered air or contaminants with the adjacent environment.

Closed System Drug-Transfer Device

A drug-transfer device that mechanically prohibits the transfer of environmental contaminants into the system and the escape of hazardous drug or vapor concentrations outside the system.

Compounding

For purposes of these guidelines, compounding simply means the mixing of ingredients to prepare a medication for patient use. This activity would include dilution, admixture, repackaging, reconstitution, and other manipulations of sterile preparations.

Controlled Area

For purposes of these guidelines, a controlled area is the area designated for preparing sterile preparations. This is referred to as the buffer zone (i.e., the clean room in which the laminar-airflow workbench is located) by USP.

Contamination

The deposition of potentially dangerous material where it is not desired, particularly where its presence may be harmful or constitute a hazard.

Cytotoxic

A pharmacologic compound that is detrimental or destructive to cells within the body.

D

Deactivation

Treating a chemical agent (such as a hazardous drug) with another chemical, heat, ultraviolet light, or other agent to create a less hazardous agent.

Decontamination

Inactivation, neutralization, or removal of toxic agents, by mechanical or chemical means.

E

Engineering Controls

Devices designed to eliminate or reduce worker exposures to chemical, biological, radiological, ergonomic, or physical hazards. Examples include laboratory fume hoods, glove bags, retracting syringe needles, sound-dampening materials to reduce noise levels, safety interlocks, and radiation shielding.

Exposure

The condition of being subjected to something, as to chemicals, that may have a harmful effect. Acute exposure is exposure of short duration, usually exposure of heavy intensity; chronic exposure is long-term exposure, either continuous or intermittent, usually referring to exposure of low intensity.

G

Genotoxic

Damaging to DNA, pertaining to agents (radiation or chemical substances) known to damage DNA, thereby causing mutations or cancer.

H

Hazardous Drug

Any drug identified by at least one of the following six criteria: carcinogenicity, teratogenicity or developmental toxicity, reproductive toxicity in humans, organ toxicity at low doses in humans or animals, genotoxicity, or new drugs that mimic existing hazardous drugs in structure or toxicity.

Hazardous Drug Spill, Contained
Hazardous drug agent in an unintended location but confined in such a manner that it cannot spread or be dispersed (e.g., liquid hazardous drug absorbed into bed linen).

Hazardous Drug Spill, Uncontained
Hazardous drug agent in an unintended location, not confined in a container or absorbent material; exists in a manner which can be spread or dispersed (e.g., liquid hazardous drug on a nonabsorbent surface, solid or powdered hazardous drug on any open surface).

Hazardous Drug Waste, Disposable
Hazardous drug, or equipment or material contaminated with a hazardous drug , which is intended for single use only (e.g., excess or unused drug solutions, hazardous drug which is no longer required, IV tubing that was used to administer a hazardous drug, absorbent towels used to clean up an uncontained hazardous drug spill).

Hazardous Drug Waste, Non-Disposable
Equipment or material contaminated with a hazardous drug but which can be successfully decontaminated for re-use (e.g., bed linens used for patients being treated with hazardous drugs, expensive devices used to prepare or administer drug solutions).

Hazardous Waste
Any waste that is a RCRA-listed hazardous waste [40 CFR 261.30–33] or that meets a RCRA characteristic of ignitability, corrosivity, reactivity, or toxicity as defined in 40 CFR 261.21–24.

High-Efficiency Particulate Air (HEPA) Filter
High-efficiency particulate air filter rated 99.97% efficient in capturing 0.3-micron-diameter particles.

Horizontal Laminar Flow Hood (Horizontal Laminar Flow Clean Bench)
A device that protects the work product and the work area by supplying HEPA-filtered air to the rear of the cabinet and producing a horizontal flow across the work area and out toward the worker.

I

Isolator (or Barrier Isolator)
A closed system made up of four solid walls, an air-handling system, and transfer and interaction devices. The walls are constructed so as to provide surfaces that are cleanable with coving between wall junctures. The air-handling system provides HEPA filtration of both inlet and exhaust air. Transfer of materials is accomplished through air locks, glove rings, or ports. Transfers are designed to minimize the entry of contamination. Manipulations can take place through either glove ports or half-suits.

M

Mutagen
A chemical or physical agent that induces or increases genetic mutations by causing changes in DNA.

P

Plenum
Space within a biohazard cabinet where air flows; plenums may either be under positive (greater than atmospheric pressure) or negative pressure,

depending on whether the air is "blown" or "sucked" through the space.

R

Respirator

Any device designed to provide the wearer with respiratory protection against inhalation of a hazardous atmosphere.

T

Trough

Drain spillage trough; an area below the biological safety cabinet's work surface, provided to retain spillage from the work area.

U

Utility Gloves

Heavy, disposable gloves, similar to household latex gloves.

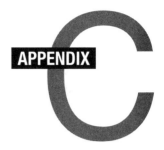

Self-Assessment Answer Key

QUESTION/ANSWER

Chapter 1

1. A
2. B
3. A
4. D
5. C

Chapter 2

1. A
2. B
3. A
4. A
5. A

Chapter 3

1. A
2. D
3. B
4. B
5. A

Chapter 4

1. A
2. B
3. A
4. A

Chapter 5

1. D
2. A
3. B
4. A
5. C

Chapter 6

1. B
2. A
3. B
4. C
5. A

Chapter 7

1. B, C
2. A
3. B
4. A
5. A

Chapter 8

1. B
2. B, C, E
3. A
4. C
5. B

Chapter 9

1. A
2. D
3. B
4. B
5. A

Index

A

R

S